Bouncing Forward

My Journey Battling
Guillain-Barré Syndrome

By Carrie Campbell Grimes

Bouncing Forward:
My Journey with Guillain-Barré Syndrome

ISBN: 978-0-578-48652-9

About the pictures: Many of the pictures taken during Carrie's journey
were snapped on cell phones with no thought they'd someday be part of a
book. Please forgive the occasional blurriness. We hope the images help you
understand Carrie's journey.

For my two biggest cheerleaders through my GBS adventure,
my husband Jeff and my older son Will.

Preface

Stop and smell the roses.

I had heard that phrase all my life, but didn't understand its wisdom until I experienced a health battle in late 2013 and throughout 2014. Now, when my adorable son wants to smell the flowers as we walk into childcare, I realize it's okay if I'm a few minutes late to my work meeting. He is more important. Stopping to enjoy the fragrance of the flowers with my two boys, Will and Zach, is what life is about.

This is a story about having the privilege of battling Guillain-Barré Syndrome (GBS). Yes, I did say "privilege." I have learned a lot during this journey, and have come to understand that you have a choice when faced with a situation like I faced: You can accept it and figure out how to move past it, or you can fall victim to it. I chose to battle GBS head-on and remain as positive as I could (most of the time). It was *not* going to beat me!

I'm going to give the story away – I get better. Throughout this journey, I believed deep down that I would, and I think that belief was essential to the speed of my recovery. Gratitude also played a huge part in my recovery. I cannot express fully how grateful I am to every person who prayed for me, sent me flowers, stopped by, or sent me an encouraging card. Every one of those people played a part in my recovery. You hear repeatedly how powerful your network of family and friends can be in your healing. In the middle of that network was my amazing husband, Jeff. He was the epicenter of my world during my battle. He was my rock, by my side ninety-five percent of the time (spending his other twenty-five percent with our son Will. Yes, he was definitely putting in more than one hundred percent while I was sick). Jeff sent emails to our friends and family throughout our journey. These emails were powerful in many ways. They created a prayer network that encapsulated me. And, for our family and friends, they offered encouragement and faith that I would get better. Each chapter will begin with one of Jeff's email updates, followed by my recollection of the details.

I have also included a chapter dedicated to the people who supported me. I wish I could also include every card, balloon, and present I received! Instead, I asked my friends and family to sit down and write what they remember about my journey with GBS. Perspectives are powerful. I want to share that power by including the unique points of view of some key people who came along with me in this battle. I hope these thoughts at the end of the book help round out the story.

I want to provide some background to the title of this book. I read the *Happiness Advantage* by Shawn Achor. One chapter mentions people who go through life-altering health events. Instead of just "bouncing back" from these health issues, the book suggests that people are "bouncing forward" as the process enriches their lives. I don't ever want to go through it again, BUT I am thankful to have survived GBS and feel like I am bouncing forward. I hope this book will help other patients and their families who are battling GBS. I also want this book to be a reminder to my son Will, my husband Jeff, and myself of the journey we endured and conquered!

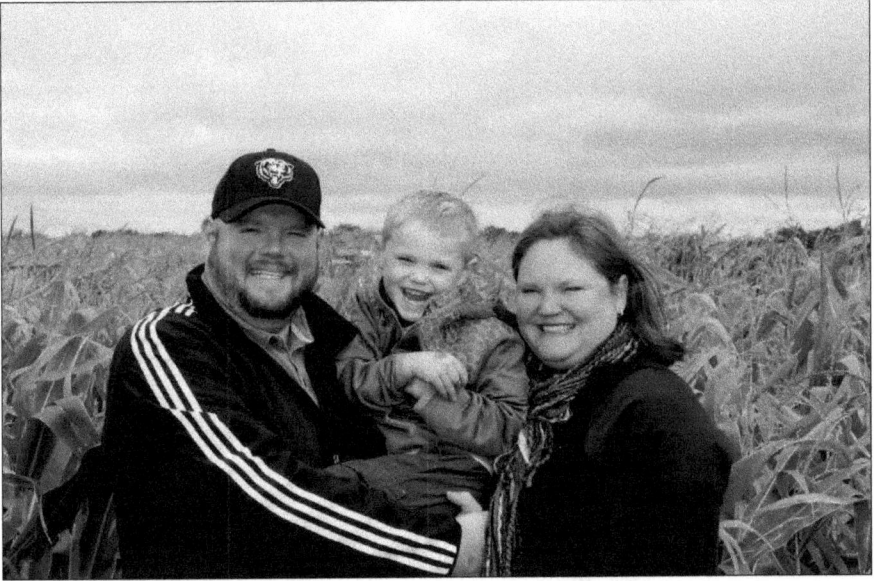

Top: *Grimes family 2013. Jeff, Will, and Carrie.*
Bottom: Grimes family 2018. Jeff, Will, Zach, and Carrie.

December 10, 2013

Tue, Dec 10, 2013 at 3:44 p.m., from Jeff's email:

Friends and Family -

We appreciate all the love and support, and we'll need it as we move forward.

Carrie had a cold that started a few weeks ago, pre-Thanksgiving. She started to feel better after getting a Z-pak for what appeared to be an upper respiratory infection, but then felt worse this past Friday. She went back to her doctor to get another antibiotic and tried to rest all day Friday and Saturday. Saturday afternoon she told me she didn't feel right, and that her hands and feet were tingly and numb. Sunday morning she felt even worse, so we headed into the ER. We spent all day Sunday in the ER, but all tests came back negative. The ER discharged us with the advice to return if the numbness/tingling got worse.

Sunday night and Monday morning the numbness and tingling was more pronounced up Carrie's arms and legs, along with a general weakness in her core. We had to slide down the stairs together because she was unsteady on her feet. After a few hours back in the ER, they admitted us to the ICU and started additional tests – CAT scan, cranial MRI, more labs. All again came back clean. The neurologist we were talking to told us it was almost certainly a neuropathic disorder, and as of today they're almost positive she has Guillain-Barré syndrome. This is a disorder where the immune system actually attacks the nervous system, causing the numbness, tingling, dizziness, unsteadiness and blurred vision she's been experiencing because of damage to the nerves.

The good news is, the doctor thinks because of her youth, the fact we caught it pretty early, and her relatively good health that we have a solid prognosis for recovery. Her symptoms appeared to plateau yesterday, and with a spinal MRI early this morning and a spinal tap just completed this afternoon, she should be starting IV treatment of immunoglobulin this afternoon or tonight. The infusion of healthy antibodies is supposed to suppress the damaging/attacking ones of her own immune system.

We don't have an exact timeframe, but the neuro doc estimated four to six weeks of therapy after the five-day treatment. If that's inpatient or outpatient will depend on how she initially responds.

Dick and Kathy (Carrie's parents) drove in from Nebraska yesterday to assist, and my parents are on emergency standby. Many of you have offered support and I promise to take you up on that as soon as we know more on the recovery process.

If you have questions, text or email is the quickest way to get me. Carrie's not ready for visitors yet, and she's not doing anything but resting and recovering.

I'll try to provide timely updates but for now I'm going to crash for a few hours. Thank you all again for your prayers, encouragement and support.

Jeff

It all started with what I thought was a cold. At Thanksgiving I started feeling blah—no energy, chills and then fever, and a runny nose. I rested and lay around most of Thanksgiving, thinking it would pass. I went back to work that next Monday but could not kick it. People started commenting that I didn't look good. (Don't you love when people say, "Wow, you really don't look good," as if you didn't already know you feel like crap?) At the end of the week I went to the doctor and he said I had an upper respiratory infection, gave me an antibiotic, and said I should feel better in five days, but if not, to give him a call. I started feeling a little better that weekend and worked on getting Christmas cards ordered and Christmas presents bought. It turned out to be a very good thing I got those done!

By the middle of the next week, I was still feeling crappy. I remember telling Jeff that this did not seem to be a normal cold. I had not felt this bad in a long time. Since the first antibiotic did not do much for me, on Friday, December 7th, I went back to the doctor's office and got a new antibiotic. I slept all day and the next day woke up with numb feet and hands. My husband looked up side effects of my antibiotic. Tingly hands and feet were listed, so we dismissed it. I lay on the couch all day while Jeff and Will decorated for Christmas. My friends will tell you that you know I am sick when I don't help decorate for Christmas! The next morning my legs felt very weak.

"I just don't feel right," I told Jeff with a quiver in my voice and tears starting to stream down my cheeks. "Something is very wrong. I think we need to go to the emergency room."

We went to Lake Forest Hospital. They ran some tests, asked me questions, then ran some more tests. We sat in the tiny emergency "room" waiting. After seven hours, the resident doctor came in, spoke with us, and left. The attending doctor came in, asked us a few questions, then he, too, disappeared. The resident came back about thirty minutes later and asked me to walk down the hall to the restroom. Walking the twenty feet was hard, and I was moving slowly, but I could walk. The resident watched me and asked me to sit back down.

"I think it's just a side effect of the antibiotic," he said, "but you could have this rare syndrome called Guillain-Barré. Come back if your symptoms get worse."

It is incredible that this resident diagnosed the GBS that early. Later, as you will learn, they ran a spinal tap that confirmed his suspicion. I often wonder how different my case of GBS might have been if they'd run the spinal tap that night and started treatment sooner. Hindsight is always twenty-twenty, right? My story wasn't meant to go that way and I do believe things happen for a reason. So off we went that night, me still feeling like total crap with what we thought was a reaction to the antibiotic. We planned to follow up with my primary care doctor the next day.

Our friends, Heather and David Bush, had come over to watch Will while we went to the hospital. We drove the fifteen minutes home, and I realized I wasn't sure I could go up the two steps into our house.

"That's silly," I thought to myself and gave it a try.

I tripped on the first step and David and Jeff had to help me up. They got me on the couch, and I lay there for a long time. Eventually Jeff convinced me we could get upstairs to bed, but it took Jeff's help to get there. I did not sleep well. I had pain in my legs and hands in addition to constant sweating. The next morning, I got up to go to the bathroom and fell to the ground. My feet were completely numb and now my legs weren't working. They were tingly and numb as well.

"Something is very wrong, and we need to go back to the hospital!" I yelled to Jeff.

I don't really remember how I got dressed but I am confident Jeff had to assist. I could not walk down the stairs, so I slid down stair by stair on my butt. When I got to the bottom, Jeff put me in a computer chair and wheeled me to the back door. Good improvisation! Jeff somehow helped me down the two stairs in to our garage and got me in the car. We then took Will to school and went back to Lake Forest Hospital. I'll never forget the intake nurse.

"Weren't you here yesterday? Aren't you supposed to just follow up with your primary care doctor? Why are you here?"

I felt horrible, but started questioning our decision to return to the hospital. When the intake nurse left for a minute I turned to Jeff and asked, "Should we go home?"

"Absolutely not!" Jeff said. Thankfully he was a voice of reason.

The same resident was there who had seen us the day before. We told him my symptoms had worsened and he had a neurologist come and see me right away. The neurologist ordered several tests and admitted me to the ICU. They ran an MRI which showed nothing. They thought maybe I had multiple sclerosis.

At this point Jeff called my parents and they got in the car mid-day to drive to Chicago from Lincoln, Nebraska – about 520 miles. It was apparent something serious was going on and we needed help to take care of Will.

In the ICU, I continued to get weaker and weaker. That first night, the nurse helped me get up to go to the bathroom. When

I finished, I tried to stand up, but my legs just gave out and I fell. I remember the nurse kept saying, "Just stand up. Push up on your legs. Come on, you can do it."

The scary thing was, I could not do it. I could not push up through my legs. I had no strength. It took six people, including two security guards, to help me back into bed. If this was a comic movie, I am sure that scene would have brought the house down; half-naked woman trying to get back in bed being lifted by two security guards, two nurses, and two male staff members. At the time I guarantee you it was not funny. I was scared. It finally hit me how serious this was.

That was the last time I got out of bed for several weeks. My legs were paralyzed.

My parents arrived Monday night and went straight to our house to take care of Will. On Tuesday it was great to see them, and their presence afforded Jeff a chance to leave the hospital for a few hours. Eventually, on Tuesday, December 10th a spinal tap confirmed that I had Guillain-Barré syndrome. With that diagnosis, they started IVIG treatment—intravenous treatment of immunoglobulin.

Treatments were scheduled five times, every other day over ten days. At first, they didn't seem to do much. By Wednesday I remember trying to drink the juice on my lunch tray. It went down the wrong pipe and I started coughing and choking. My mom had to feed me lunch. I could not raise my arm off the bed. I thought I was just tired, worn out. In reality, the nerve damage was progressing up my body. My arms were becoming paralyzed and the nerves around my lungs were also starting to be affected.

They took me down for a swallow test. It was not fun, but then again, most health tests are not the definition of fun. After

I swallowed a liquid that tasted disgusting, they watched on x-ray to see if the fluid or food was going down the right pipe. I could see the fluid going down the wrong pipe as I started coughing. The test confirmed my nerves and muscles were so weakened, I had to go on a diet of thickened liquids.

December 12, 2013

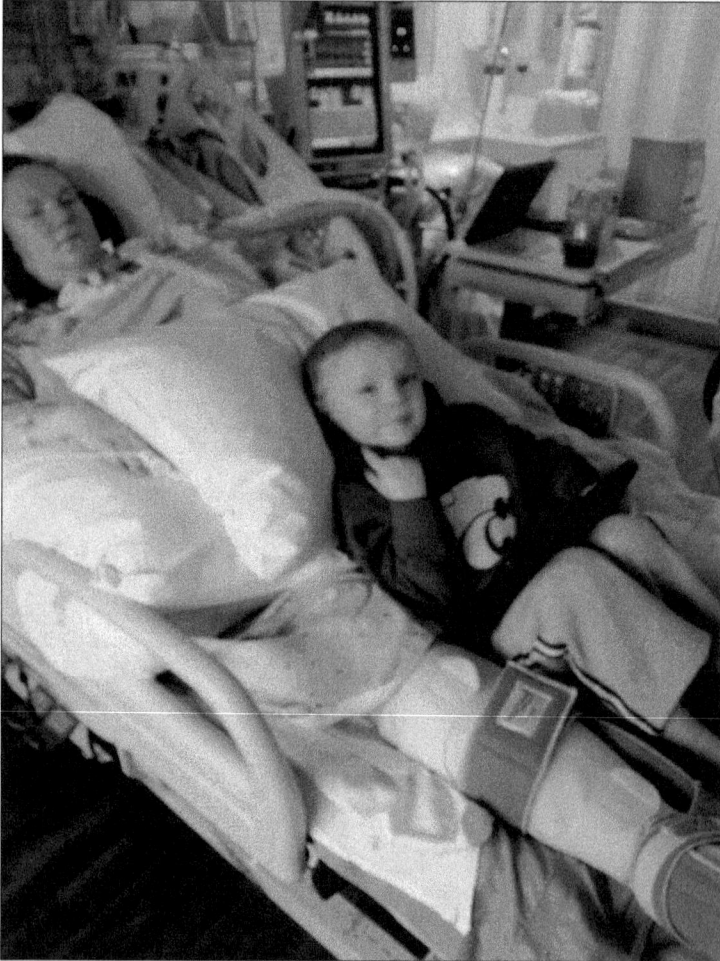

Will visiting the hospital and sitting with Mom.

Thu, Dec 12, 2013 at 8:12 p.m., from Jeff's email:

Update for Thursday

The last couple days have been up and down. We thought we'd hit the 'plateau' of symptoms no longer progressing, but last night Carrie had real trouble sleeping, waking up gasping for air and sweating profusely. Today the neurologist made the decision to transfer Carrie to the downtown Northwestern Memorial Hospital. Her lung 'vital capacity' had steadily decreased until today it was under 750mL, where a normal adult's should be a couple liters. She has had three of the IVIG treatments and thus far they have not done much. Her muscles that support her lungs have started to become compromised, so she is now intubated. The way it was explained to me is that she's doing all the breathing on her own, but the machine just helps her lungs expand to take in more oxygen. She is lightly sedated just to keep her relaxed while she acclimates to the tubes and is resting comfortably now. Hopefully we both get some much-needed sleep tonight.

We'll know more about the treatment plan tomorrow from the head doctor. I've heard many stories from friends and family about knowing people who have experienced this syndrome or similar and have recovered fully. Carrie had an opportunity today to speak directly to someone who had this disease and came through with no lingering side effects. We are staying positive and glad that we've moved to the best neuro docs in Illinois. I'm already about 500% more impressed with the nurses and residents I've met this evening.

Sorry for the delayed reporting, the last couple of days seem like a blur. Dick and Kathy have been rock solid and Mr. Will was able to see mommy tonight and give her a kiss and tell her he loved her.

Jeff

By the morning of Thursday, December 12th, my breathing was becoming more difficult, so the neurologist said she would like to transfer me downtown to Northwestern (NW) Memorial Hospital (NMH) as they had more experience and tools to help me. She feared the paralysis was going to spread to my lungs and require intubation. The Northwestern downtown campus would be a safer place for me.

While waiting for the transfer, the Chaplin stopped by. She said a very nice prayer for me and my mom. I spent some time talking to her about what I was experiencing. Once she found out I had GBS she started telling us about a gentleman who worked with her in the hospital who had recovered from the syndrome. She wanted me to meet him to see there was hope. Since we were leaving shortly, she bolted out to find him. Twenty minutes later, this man came by my room holding a prayer shawl. He gave it to me and said it was from the Chaplin. He went on to tell me his story. He shared how his paralysis spread and how weak he was. It took time, but he recovered. I asked him if he walked out of the hospital.

"Yes, with a walker," he answered, "but then I continued to get stronger."

He had almost fully recovered after a year. He said if he was really tired his feet may hurt or feel numb, but most days he felt back to normal. It was tremendously helpful to meet someone who had gotten through GBS, especially right before I continued to go downhill. Hope is what I had to hold onto throughout this journey. Positive energy, positive thinking – I will get better. I am so glad that Jeff and the doctors chose not to tell me the negative statistics, the probability of some of my issues. Per the National Institute of Neurological Disorders and Stroke, "Guillain-Barré syndrome can be a devastating disorder because of its sudden and rapid, unexpected onset of weakness—and usually actual paralysis. Fortunately, seventy percent of people with GBS eventually experience full recovery. With careful intensive care and successful treatment of infection, autonomic dysfunction and other medical complications, even those individuals with respiratory failure usually survive.

"The recovery period may be as little as a few weeks up to a few years. Some individuals still report ongoing improvement after two years. About thirty percent of those with Guillain-Barré have residual weakness after three years. About fifteen percent of individuals experience long-term weakness; some may require ongoing use of a walker, wheelchair, or ankle support. Muscle strength may not return uniformly."

My case was in the worst five percent of cases the doctors had seen. They were telling Jeff I may not recover. They told him I might never walk again. I needed to hear that most people recover. I needed hope and reassurance which Jeff and others gave me.

"You should be able to walk again."

"It will take time, but you will get better."

"Will is doing fine."

"Will misses you but sends kisses."

"You can do this."

I was determined that my recovery was going to be successful. I was determined to be in the top five percent of recovery cases! Positive thinking helped me get better. I am confident of that.

About 1:30 p.m. the ambulance team arrived to take me downtown. We had everything packed up and ready to go. My breathing was becoming more difficult. The ambulance team got me on the gurney and strapped me in. I was getting hot and anxious (anxiety is common in GBS patients) as all of this was happening. I had only been in the hospital once in my lifetime, to deliver my son Will via C-section. So, ambulances, gurneys, breathing tests, it was all new to me.

They wheeled me downstairs and got me loaded in the ambulance, my mom in the front seat, but wouldn't you know it, the ambulance wouldn't start! I remember thinking "Are you kidding me?" So, they wheeled me back into the hospital and placed me in the emergency room area. I started to sweat more and my breathing became labored. Then I started to hyperventilate. The same resident who had admitted me happened to be in the emergency room and came over to help. They tried to calm me down and when they had difficulties doing that, they sent me back up to the ICU.

Once back in the ICU, they calmed me down. But when the new ambulance crew arrived, I could tell they were on edge.

"We are not taking her unless you can assure us she is going to make it," one of the drivers said.

Make it? What did he mean by that? Was I going to die? I started breathing very quickly again and my mind was racing.

The doctors had prepared me and my family that if the paralysis continued to spread up my body that I would most likely need to be intubated. The ambulance drivers were not confident I would make it downtown before I needed to be intubated. We had only a small window for the transfer. The ICU physician assured them I was fine and she would show them via a breathing test. They had me blow into a Spirometer to show my vital lung capacity. I passed and the next thing I knew I was on a new gurney and we were on our way. The physician told them they had one hour to get me downtown.

By now it was four p.m. on a Thursday. We had to travel fifty plus miles to reach downtown Chicago during the worst traffic day of the week. Jeff and my dad were in their cars ready to follow the ambulance.

When my mom hopped in, the ambulance driver turned to her and said, "Mom, how do you feel about lights and sirens?"

With lights on we drove down the median and shoulder of Interstate 94. We arrived downtown in just over fifty minutes. Amazing!

They got me upstairs to the neuro ICU and I was greeted by many nurses and doctors who immediately started doing tests. They asked my mom to go to the waiting room. Within ten minutes of arriving I remember having difficulty breathing. They tried a few things before discussing the need to intubate with me. I agreed. I was just so tired from trying hard to breathe.

They put me under (thank goodness) and put in an orotracheal, a tube in my mouth through to the trachea. I remember the doctor telling me that if I woke up and could not handle having the tubes in my mouth, they would sedate me. Jeff says I woke up three different times and freaked out before I finally could handle having the trach tube and a feeding tube in my mouth.

I never intended to move in, but I became a resident of ICU Room 810. The next few days are a blur as they kept me sedated. They had decided to finish the last two IVIG treatments then determine a course of action if those did not work. I was on painkillers and sedatives to keep me calm. Jeff spent the night with me, which was so reassuring.

People often ask how I spent my days while in the hospital. The first month or so, I slept, sometimes stared at the TV, and often just lay in my bed thinking. My brain was never affected by the GBS, so while my body was shutting down around me, my mind was wide awake. I think I wrote my employees' end-of-year performance reviews ten times over in my brain. It was so frustrating, though, because at this point, I could not talk due to the tubes in my mouth. I could not hold a phone or iPad. My hands and arms were paralyzed. I could not watch TV for long periods of time, as my blurry vision would cause me to get headaches.

Someone in the hospital, a speech therapist or nurse, brought a communication chart for me to use. I could still blink with one eye, so if I wanted to tell my parents, or Jeff or a friend anything I had to use this board. They would point to a letter and if I blinked, they would know it was correct. This was a tedious process and most of us didn't have a ton of patience. Whomever I was "speaking" to would get the first letter of a word from me and start guessing words. My dad, Dick, was notorious for doing this. If he pointed to the letter A and I blinked, he didn't wait for the next letter. He'd just yell, "Aardvark!"

Yes – that is exactly what I was looking for in the hospital dad, an aardvark!

A few weeks later, once I could communicate a little better, I realized I had to laugh at the situation, but in the moment, if I could have rolled my eyes at him… I would have.

The communication board helped for sure. At moments my family got glimpses of my funny side, but most of the time I would get irritated when I was trying to spell something. For example, I would spell out three letters, meaning I would have waited for them to put their finger on the letter I wanted, blink fast, and then we would move on to the next letter. By the fourth or fifth letter they would often forget what the first three letters were. Annoying? Ummm yes! I finally convinced my family they could write the letters/words on the white board in my room as I spelled them. They also realized there were some key words I spelled a lot, like H-O-T.

I was hot all the time! You will get tired of me telling you throughout this story that I was extremely hot. With GBS, because your nerves have lost the myelin sheathing, they don't connect with your brain, so your body is all whacked out. In most cases, this causes people to be extremely hot all the time. When they put cold washcloths on my forehead, within a few minutes it would be scalding hot! In the ICU, they had a cooling blanket they laid underneath me. It was like having a water bed underneath me that was as cold as a snowy mountain when you fall down skiing. It felt so good! After a few minutes, my body temperature would start dropping, I would get the shivers and ask them to turn the cooling blanket off. Then I would start getting hot again. It was a vicious cycle of me using the letter board to tell whomever was in the room to call the nurse. Then that person calling the nurse to turn the blanket on, then calling the nurse to turn it off. Eventually the nurses taught Jeff how to operate the cooling blanket. I missed that blanket when I moved to the rehab hospital. If I could have taken it with me, it would have saved a lot of wet washcloth preparations by my family and friends.

Other words I often spelled.

T-V. Even though my vision was blurry, I would sometimes want the TV on for the noise, or to watch something to allow my brain some time to rest. College football bowl games were on almost every day so that helped keep my mind distracted! Even though my alma mater, Purdue University, hadn't produced a solid team since the Drew Brees era, I enjoyed having football on to pass some time.

J-E-F-F. I wanted Jeff by my side at all times. When I would get anxious, I felt he was the one person who understood what I needed. He knew how to comfort me or calm me. The tough thing was he barely got any sleep the month of December. Whenever he would leave the hospital, it seemed like something went wrong, so my mom had to call and have him come back. He earned his husband stripes!

W-A-T-E-R. I asked for water a lot. And the crummy thing was, I could not drink water for more than a month. Because my muscles were weak and the nerves were not connecting to my brain properly, the swallowing refluxes were not working right so the last thing they wanted to give me were liquids that could go down the wrong pipe in my trachea and put water in my lungs. That could lead to pneumonia. Still, I asked for water all the time. I craved water. People asked me if I was hungry and what foods I desired. I was not hungry at all. Food was not even appealing, but water…I dreamt about drinking water. It was like I was in the desert and would see mirages of water. It makes me thirsty just recalling how badly I wanted to drink water.

W-I-L-L. I wanted updates on my little guy often. He was three and a half when this all began and was a trooper through it all. Kids are resilient, and Will proved to be no different. He would come visit and would sit on my hospital bed with me. It was killing me to miss out on his daily routine. I was sad not to hear him tell me about his school day and what he had for lunch and his silly stories at the dinner table. Will and Jeff were the two biggest reasons I fought so hard to get better.

One of my best friends, Laura Janitz, and I still chuckle about the first time she came to the hospital and my dad wanted to teach her how to use the communication board. He was so excited to show Laura how they had figured out a way to "talk" with me.

"Go ahead and ask her a question," he said.

I honestly have no idea what question Laura asked, but my dad was proudly holding the board. I paused and my dad started to move his finger on the letters on the board. My eyes looked confused, they said. I tried to move my eyes from side to side. I was willing my head to move, but nothing. Dad kept moving his finger and I didn't blink my eye. My dad, confused, started over. I blinked on the letter B, then I blinked on the letter A then on C. A little while longer... K.

"BACK!" they shouted, and started worrying that my back hurt, or that I wanted to move back, or that something was wrong with my gown in the back.

"NO!!!!!!!!!!!!!!" I was trying to shout, but no one could hear me or tell how extremely agitated I was. I finally got them to go back to the board. W... A... R... D... BACKWARD? Laura, my dad, and my mom spent another five minutes trying to figure out what I wanted them to do. Did I want to face another way? Did I want them to move back?

All of a sudden Laura said, "Dick, are you holding the card backwards?"

"YESSSSSSSSSSSSSSSSSSS!!!!!" I wanted to shout. Finally.

The entire time he had held the communication board backwards, so I had to try to read letters backwards! Let me tell you how hard that is when you are dizzy and your vision is fuzzy. They all had a good chuckle. I think I decided to take a nap to calm my frustration.

December 14, 2013

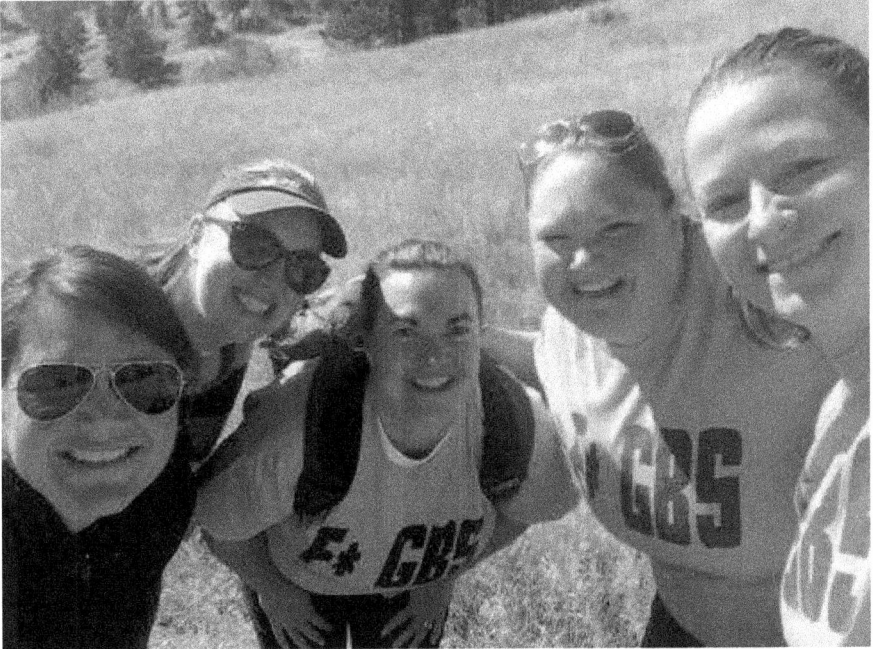

Carrie's amazing friends—BACH (Jennifer, Brooke, Patty, Carrie and Laura).

Sat, Dec 14, 2013 at 9:30 P.M., from Jeff's email:

Update for Saturday, December 14th

Carrie had the fifth treatment of IV immunoglobulin today. She has not yet started to respond to the treatment—still having loss of control, tingling and numbness in all her limbs. She's really frustrated by not being able to communicate by anything other than spelling words out from a list via nods and blinks. Her doctor told us today that there is still a long road ahead. We are hoping to see some turnaround this week—if the IVIG is doing its work, her antibodies should stop attacking her nervous system and the initial inflammation should go down. At that point, we'll know more about what kind of rehab we are looking at by how quickly she can recover some function.

Carrie would enjoy (and was recommended by her doctor) for folks to call her and talk to her. Any day, any time she's awake I'll try to have her phone ringer on. Wednesday is her birthday and I'm sure she would love a call from you. I've read her all your supportive emails and texts and she and I both appreciate all of the love and support.

She is still in the ICU and likely will be through this week. This means no flowers or anything can be sent to the room, but if you can swing by, she can have brief visits. My folks arrived today and will be taking care of Will in Libertyville this week, so my plan is to be downtown all week - either at the hospital or crashing in Jeff and Brooke's spare bedroom.

Jeff

"Will I get better?"

I remember asking the neurologist that question. Of course, they cannot promise anything, but he would say, "Most people recover from GBS. It just takes time."

The doctors would make rounds each morning in the ICU. All six or seven or ten of them, depending on how many interns were there, would shuffle over next to my bed. I felt like I was in an episode of *Grey's Anatomy* or *House*. Doctors would present my case and would then ask me to squeeze their fingers. I would intensely scrunch my face up (but my face was paralyzed too), and my brain would be telling my fingers to squeeze, but there was nothing. The doctors would then put their hands on the bottom of my feet and ask me to push. Again, I would squeeze my eyes shut and visualize pushing with all my might, but neither my foot nor my leg did anything. These tests became a depressing morning ritual that took a toll on my morale.

A few times when it was just Jeff and me in the room, I would ask, "Am I going to get better? Will I ever be able to walk again?"

I was scared, anxious, and fearful of how our lives had changed so quickly. Jeff was a saint. He would be the positive one, the cheerleader, encouraging me that I was going to get better. The ironic thing was that I had always been the optimist in our relationship. Jeff tended to be the realist, telling me when the glass was half empty. Roles reversed for us during my GBS journey. Jeff became the optimist, giving me the positive energy and vibes that I needed to pull through. This was tough on Jeff, because he was the one talking to the doctors outside of my room. He was the one carrying the burden of "fearing the worst" for both of us, and he hid it well.

Many months after those initial weeks in the ICU, once Jeff knew I was on a path to recovery, he opened up about those first few weeks.

"I was scared to death. The doctors told me that you may never get off the ventilator. They prepared me mentally for the worst that could happen. They explained to me how our lives would change. The doctors told me, 'Carrie's case of GBS is very extreme and although most people recover, it may not be the case for Carrie. She may never walk again.'"

I was shocked. That was a lot to shoulder. I asked Jeff whom he talked to through all of this. The first week or so he kept this information to himself so he wouldn't worry my parents or my friends. Then he started talking with his parents, Greg and Ardie. They offered him an outlet where he could share the scary doomsday news, then put on the positive, motivating face for me.

I saw a psychologist while I was in the NMH ICU. She was a very kind woman who always made me feel comfortable and safe when I was talking to her. Mentally I was doing okay, but not great. The worst part was the anxiety, especially in regard to my breathing. I was also having trouble sleeping. Not only was I waking up in the middle of the night unable to get back to sleep, but when I woke, I often thought there were people in my room. I remember waking Jeff up and spelling out P-E-O-P-L-E on the communication board. Eventually he figured out that I was hallucinating, and I thought there were other people in my room. I also woke Brooke, one of my best friends since college, one night telling her the same thing. I remember her convincing me that we were the only people in the room, as she ran her fingers through my hair, just as I do with Will when he is trying to fall asleep. My friends took care of me as if I was their own child or mother.

I am extremely lucky to have a core group of women friends who were always by my side when Jeff could not be there. This group had gone on vacation together every year since we graduated college. We call ourselves BACH based on our maiden names (Ball and Becker, Anderson, Campbell, and Hemingway). We have been through many exciting moments (weddings, childbirth) and some tough times, and my friends rallied during this difficult time in my life to help pull me through.

I also woke up multiple nights convinced they had moved me into a new room. Nope, I was in room 810 the entire time. I think the combination of the medications coupled with the anxiety of GBS caused my brain to believe I was in a new room. Hallucinations became a normal occurrence.

Unfortunately, I did not have the ability to push the nurse call button. They brought in some other gadgets they thought may work for me. One was a really, really big button they put on my neck where I had a little functionality. I would try to press it between my cheek and shoulder, but it didn't work. I was not strong enough yet. So, while in the hospital I was unable to call anyone if I was having difficulties. I can tell you, that tends to add to a person's anxiety. The good news is that most of the time Jeff was with me and really eased my anxiety. But poor Jeff. He could not be there every day, twenty-four hours a day for weeks on end. Thank God for the friends who would come and give Jeff a few hours of respite.

But when Jeff or my friends were sleeping, I could not make any noise or move anything to wake them up. We brainstormed a bunch of ideas and eventually landed on the jingle bells. It was a Christmas ornament a friend had given me years ago that had a red rope about six inches long with a bell on each end. They would set the bells on my shoulder (the only area of my body I could move) and I would try to jingle the bells. It worked about fifty percent of the time. The other half of the time I could not muster enough energy to make the bells jingle, or the nurses would come in to give me medicine or turn me (something they did every two hours) and they would take the bells off my shoulder and forget to put them back.

"Put my bells back where you found them! Santa says!" I would be shouting on the inside, but no one could hear me. I would try to get the nurses to get the communication board and spell out B-E-L-L-S but that hardly ever worked either. I think they just thought I was losing my bells.

If I tried to communicate with the nurse long enough, it would usually wake up Jeff or Brooke or Laura, and then I would spell B-E-L-L and they would explain to the nurse they had to keep the bells on my shoulder. The nurses meant well – they were all very friendly—but they had so much work to do, they often forgot those details. I loved it when I had the same nurse two days in a row. My anxiety would decrease so much because that nurse had worked with me and understood my needs a little better. It was so hard when we had new nurses and had to "train" them to my idiosyncrasies.

December 16, 2013

Carrie and her good friend Kathy.

Mon, Dec 16, 2013 at 10:22 P.M., from Jeff's email:

Update for Monday, December 16th

Carrie had a small breakthrough last night—she felt more able to control her fingers on the iPad. This morning both she and her doctor agreed that she was weaker in her neck and head, so we've started a new treatment. The IVIG has had time to work and has not shown appreciable recovery yet. Carrie had a large-bore IV put into her neck just before noon today and then we started plasmapheresis tonight, pulling out her blood and replacing the plasma in it, then pumping it back in. This obviously has a larger impact on her body, so she is very tired and achy now.

I have been reading every email and text to her, all of the Facebook posts I've seen, and I put all her voicemails on speakerphone. We had several visitors over the weekend and today and I know she enjoyed seeing and hearing from every one of you. Listening to your words of encouragement and stories is the best part of her day.

Jeff

Throughout my time in the hospital, I honestly did not feel good at all. I was in pain from the nerves trying to regrow and reconnect. I cannot describe that throbbing and dull pain – it is a mix of cramps, childbirth, and a sprained ankle all wrapped into one. I also was so hot all the time, I was uncomfortable. I could not move myself or shift in bed, so I was quite often agitated. Imagine lying in the same position for two hours – you would become easily disgruntled.

Sleep was a challenge. I would usually take some of my medications around 8:00 or 9:00 p.m. and fall asleep for a few hours. Then I would wake up around 1:00 or 2:00 a.m. and be unable to go back to sleep. Sometimes it would be because my mind was racing – thinking about what I was missing at home with Will and Jeff, angry I was experiencing this, or worrying about how much work had piled up while I was out sick. And I was scared. Would I recover from this? Would I be able to hold my son again? Would I ever be able to walk? I lay awake many nights in the ICU running through all of these thoughts over and over again. Since my mind was fully functioning but my body was not cooperating, it felt like my brain went into overdrive, trying to solve any issue or problem I could come up with. The dilemma was that my brain could not will my muscles and nerves to work.

There is nothing worse than not being able to sleep. Your body needs sleep to recover, to heal. Jeff, my parents and my friends would try to convince me I should get more rest and try to sleep. I totally understood what they were saying, but since I could not talk it was very hard to communicate all the thoughts going through my head, the fear that woke me up multiple times a night, and the anxiety I felt.

Brooke spent some of those nights with me. Brooke and her husband Jeff were lifesavers for us. Our friendships go back many years. Brooke and I met during sorority rush, and although I thought she was an angry bitch the first day I met her, we ended up both being selected to join the Tri-Delta sorority and quickly became best friends. We have lived together, traveled together, and been a red-headed duo for more than twenty years. Jeff Roberts met my husband Jeff when they worked together in Lincoln, Nebraska. We like to think we helped play matchmakers to start Brooke and Jeff Anderobertses' love story.

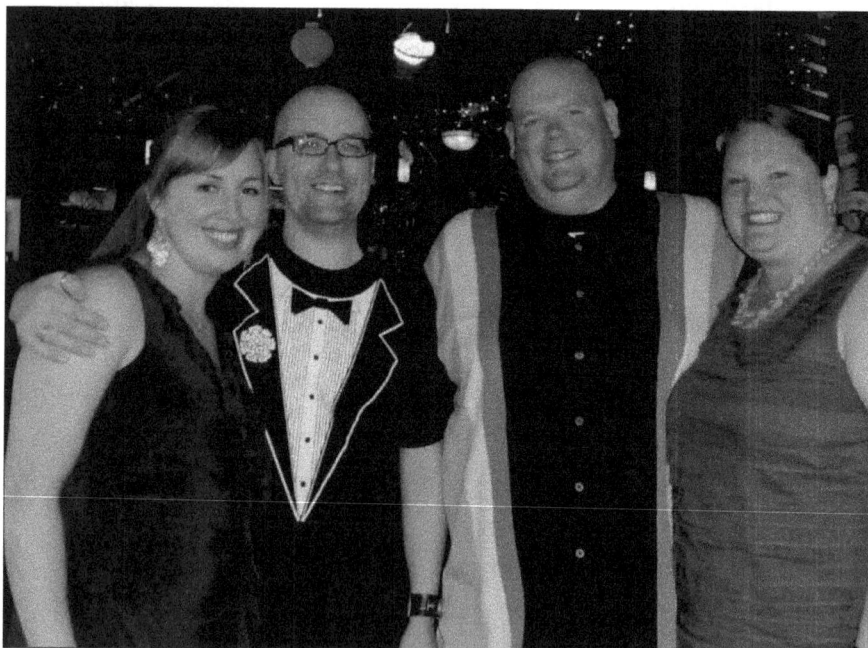

Brooke, Jeff, Jeff and Carrie. Jeff and Brooke were amazing friends during Carrie's battle with GBS.

Many nights, my husband Jeff stayed at the Anderobertses' condo building where he could sleep in a real bed. The condo was only ten minutes from the hospital, so he could return quickly in case something happened. This was so much better than being more than fifty miles away in Libertyville where our home was.

Brooke was wonderful at finding ways to make me more comfortable. To try to help me sleep better, she would give me a massage and play classical music. Everybody did what they could to make me comfortable, but the reality was I was in such pain and so consumed by fear, that sleep still eluded me.

I also now think I woke up at 2:00 a.m. because I knew bath time occurred between four and five, and I hated sponge baths. Don't get me wrong, I wanted to be as clean as I could, but sponge baths meant they were going to roll me in my bed. Basically they had to "log roll" me because I could not move any of my paralyzed body parts. When they did this, my heart rate would often skyrocket, causing the monitors to beep uncontrollably, causing my heart rate to go up even more. It was also extremely painful. Even though I could not move my legs and arms, it hurt to be touched or moved. Any slight touch felt as if I had pins and needles and throbbing all mixed together on that body part. Imagine how it feels when your foot falls asleep, then multiply that by 1000. That is how my entire body felt if someone touched me. Since I couldn't talk or make a lot of facial expressions, it was difficult to communicate that pain to nurses or family members. I ended up absorbing that pain internally, which often escalated my anxiety. So I would lay awake watching the hands of the clock move, willing them to stop before bath time.

December 18, 2013 was my thirty-sixth birthday. What a fun way to spend your birthday, huh? Two good friends came into town for the occasion. Kathy Lunzmann came from Nebraska, and Patty Carmichael came from Michigan. A few weeks back, I had planned an awesome birthday dinner with friends at a new restaurant. Those plans got thrown out the window. I remember feeling so bad that I wasn't myself. Each morning I kept hoping I would wake up able to move my finger or a toe, or at least smile. At this point, I had no idea how long I would actually spend recovering from GBS. Though I kept thinking "I'll be better in the morning," it just doesn't work that way. Your body takes lots of time to regrow that myelin sheathing on your nerves. A very, very long time. So on my birthday, I tried to put on a happy face, or at least not show my pain as much. It was exhausting work.

I slept on and off most of the day and then I had some fun visitors come from work: Tina, Heather, Lizelle, Lauren, and others I know I am forgetting (and I apologize), but I felt so cruddy. They were all so sweet to drive down to see me, bring me gifts, wear silly hats and mustaches. And it made me happy, but honestly, I struggled to show that happiness because I was in pain. I felt like crap. I wanted to talk to my friends, but couldn't. I wanted to tell them I would be okay because I could tell when they walked into that ICU room, they were shocked by how sick I was. I had my feeding tube and my ventilator tube going through my nose and mouth at this point. I was pale as a sheet and could make no facial expressions. I was not the Carrie Campbell Grimes they knew and loved. I was someone else in a hospital bed. But they were all there to support me and show their love and that was huge for me. So it made me feel really bad when I asked them all to leave. I thought I was going to throw up or pass out or scream in pain (if I could have screamed). I needed to be alone with just Jeff and my family who I knew would not be sad if I did all of those things. I didn't want to let my friends down.

December 19, 2013

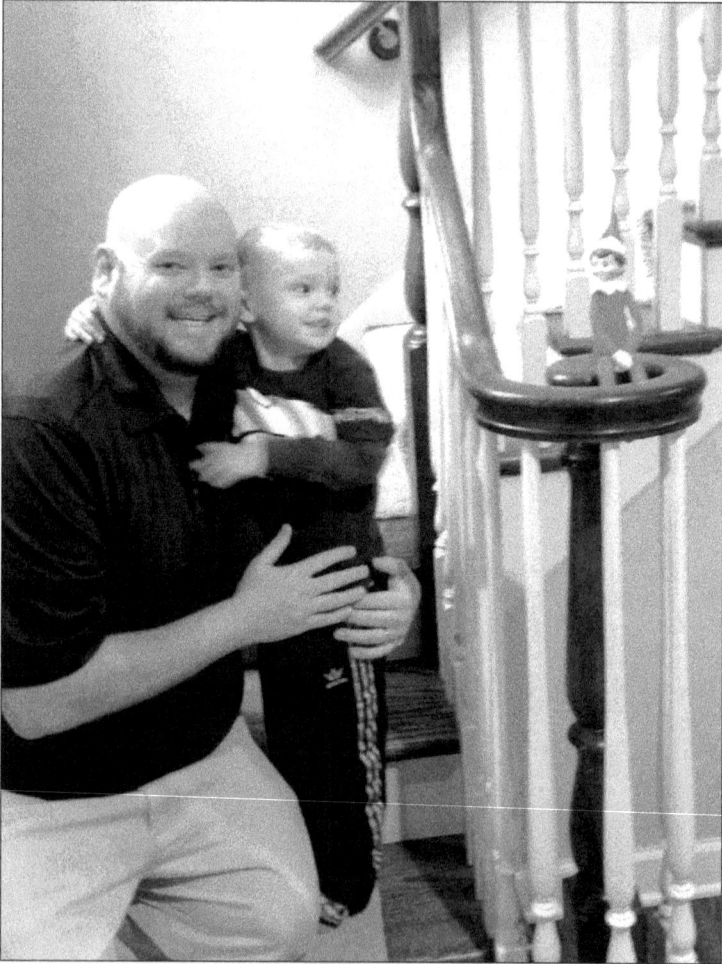

Jeff, Will, and Fred the Elf. Jeff trying to keep some normalcy for Will during Carrie's battle.

Thu, Dec 19, 2013 at 5:26 P.M., from Jeff's email:

Update for Thursday, December 19th

First off — thank you thank you thank you to everyone who came, sent emails, videos, cards and just the sheer volume of love and support for Carrie. She had about as great of a birthday as possible in the ICU. There were so many emails and videos and pictures that we haven't even shown them all to her yet! That's good because it'll give us something to do over the weekend and keep her mind busy.

She had her second plasmapheresis treatment yesterday which she completed like a champ. This morning she and the doctor both agreed that she is slowly regaining some strength, noticeably in her fingers, arms and eyelids/facial muscles. That makes three days in a row with no decline, and two in a row with improvement so the doctors are feeling confident we've got this thing on its heels.

That being said, there's still a long road to full recovery. She'll still probably be in the ICU for at least another week. Her plasmapheresis treatments are scheduled to go through Tuesday/Christmas Eve, and depending on muscle recovery for breathing and swallowing, we may be staying longer. So today she had minor surgery for a tracheostomy (breathing tube directly to throat) and direct stomach line for feeding. The advantage to these is now her mouth and nose are entirely clear of tubes so we can see her beautiful face. They also reduce the chances of inflammation and infection from the original breathing and feeding tubes.

I'll send another update soon, but know that we appreciate all of the love and support...

Jeff

By this point I was on a feeding tube, breathing machine and had a full tracheostomy. Normal life, as I knew it, was long gone. Many parts of the ICU are fuzzy for me. Jeff has since shared with me how heavily sedated they had me. He said I was conscious, but I was not myself at all. They kept me under enough sedation so that I was not extremely uncomfortable. Jeff told me prior to the surgeries to make my tubes more permanent, I would often wake up irritated and try to pull the feeding tube and breathing tubes out. I have learned that this is very normal, but still, in the moment it seemed like hell. Tubes in my nose, my mouth, and monitors beeping all the time. Many times, people told me, "The hardest place in the world to sleep is the ICU."

This nightmare I was living was not going to end soon. It was bad enough I missed my birthday, but I started to realize I would not be going home for Christmas. I would not be there on Christmas morning when Santa delivered all the cool toys we had bought Will. I started to worry about who would wrap Will's presents or how I was going to buy something for Jeff. I remember spelling out words to my parents on the communication board.

C-H-R-I-S-T-M-A-S.

P-R-E-S-E-N-T-S.

W-I-L-L.

W-R-A-P-P-ING P-A-P-E-R.

B-A-S-E-M-E-N-T C-L-O-S-E-T.

S-A-N-T-A.

P-L-E-A-S-E.

T-H-A-N-K Y-O-U.

J-E-F-F? N-O P-R-E-S-E-N-T.

They assured me they could wrap all of Will's presents and would split them up between Santa and Jeff and me. We worked out a plan so Jeff and I could watch Will on Christmas morning via Skype, then my parents said they would bring Will down to see me. Good thing I'm such a Type A person and had already bought all of Will's gifts. The bad news was I had shipped most of them to Nebraska because that is where we had planned to travel for the holidays to see both our families. So, my parents had to go home to Nebraska for a few days to get the presents I had shipped for Will and our families. Best laid plans…

Christmas is my favorite time of the year. I could not believe I was stuck in a hospital bed, unable to move, talk, roll over, or even smile.

"What a crummy deal," I kept thinking. It was hard. Many a tear was shed thinking about what I was missing. My team's holiday gathering, my birthday dinner, time off to spend with family over Christmas, presents! Unwrapping gifts, making Chex mix with my mom, Christmas dinner, seeing Will's face on Christmas morning in person and absorbing his excitement. Looking back I am still sad I missed those moments, but I am also so grateful I will get to enjoy many more Christmases in the future. There were a few nights that my situation got really bad and life-threatening and we were not sure I would see another Christmas.

One of those nights was December 19th. Heather was our ICU nurse and we loved her. She was full of energy, extremely helpful and very diligent. I was having a rough night as I just did not have the energy to breathe deeply. My heart rate kept dropping lower. The machines would all go off and Heather would rush in. It continued to happen more frequently.

Heather instructed my mom and friends who were in the room to help.

"All of you, I need you to talk to Carrie about something she is very interested in. We need to get her heart rate up!"

There were "ummms" and "ahhhhs" as everybody wracked their brains. Then I think it was Brooke who broke the silence.

"Carrie, you are not going to believe what is happening on *Scandal* (my favorite show on television at the time!)"

She went on to tell me some of the big updates on the show. The good news is I didn't remember her telling me this so it was still a surprise when I could watch TV and catch up on the episodes I missed. The great news is my heart rate started going up, and, they said I even moved one side of my lips up in a semi-smile. Heather clapped and said "Good job! Keep talking. And Carrie – keep breathing big breaths, deep breaths!" My heart rate came back into normal range.

December 21, 2013

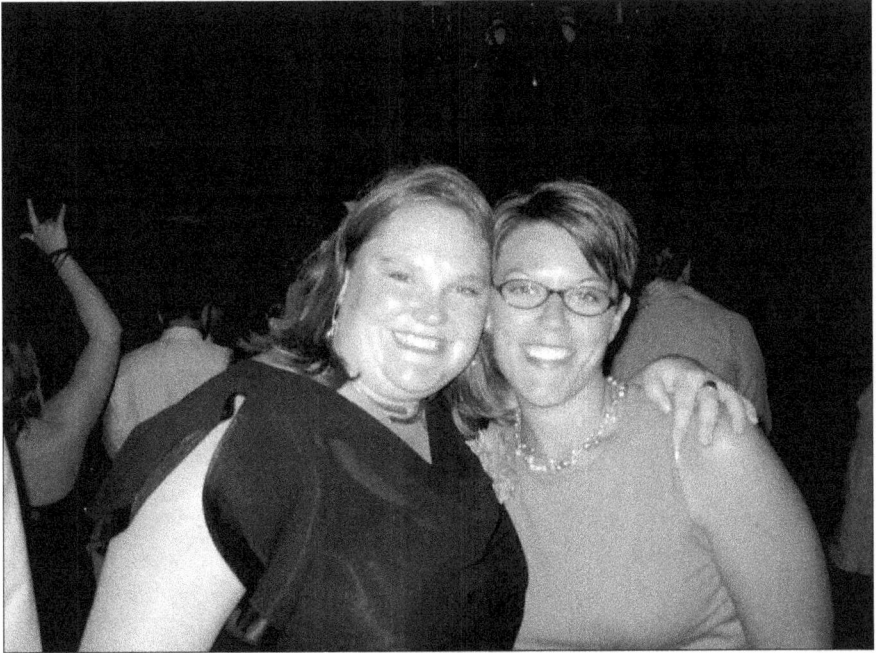

Carrie and her good friend Stephanie "Shipley."

Sat, Dec 21, 2013 at 9:02 P.M., from Jeff's email:

Update for Saturday, December 21st

Friday was a day of good progress. We tried to heal up and rest from our two surgeries. We also had a plasmapheresis treatment, which really wears her out. The neuro and respiratory doctors decided that we needed to try weaning off of the ventilator, so Friday afternoon they backed the settings down and Carrie started to do some of the breathing on her own. She did well at first, but when I went home to hang out with Will and take him to see Santa, she had a rough night. She gets very anxious when she has any trouble breathing at all – obviously if that's about the only thing you can control and it's not doing what you want it would be a little scary. So Friday night she didn't sleep well partly due to breathing anxiety and partly due to her mind racing. Saturday morning she had a little bleeding around the trach incision that went on most of the day.

When I came back Saturday afternoon there was a big group of nurses in her room. They'd rolled her over and she'd held her breath, causing all sorts of alarms and things, which of course made her more anxious. When she calmed down, she told them that she felt like it was really hard to breathe. She'd been doing most of the breathing work off ventilator for twenty-four hours, so the docs made the decision to put her more fully back onto the machine in order to get her better rest. It's a fine line of trying to get her body back doing what it needs to, versus keeping her in good shape for plasma treatments and healing up from surgeries.

Sunday we have another plasmapheresis scheduled along with standard doctor rounds. Carrie told me tonight that she appreciates the visitors, but they really wear her out and she'd like to postpone them until she's a little more stable, finished with treatments, and not working to wean off the ventilator. Keep the emails and texts and voicemails coming however, those I can share with her when she's not resting. Thank you.

Jeff

Having visitors in the hospital is tough. You want to see your friends and family, but you are also at your worst. You look horrible, feel horrible, and have zero energy. I am the kind of person who likes to entertain, tell stories, and make people feel welcome. That is hard to do when you cannot talk or smile. And it's hard on your guests. Friends and family visiting me had no idea what to expect, and when they walked into my room, I could tell many were shocked by my condition. They had read the emails from Jeff and knew I would not be myself, but I don't think most people were prepared for how sick I really was and how little I could do. The other awkward thing is that a hospital room is not meant for people who are shy about their bodies or bodily fluids. I had a feeding tube hooked up to the two cal (the 2000 Caloric diet liquid) "food" they were feeding me. I am not a bashful or modest person, just ask my friends. They tell stories all the time of me walking from the shower to my room at our sorority house in a short robe probably showing off more than the normal person. But not everyone is that bold or forward, so I felt myself being more self-conscious when people came to visit the hospital.

Two of the most interesting visitors I had while in the hospital came on Saturday, December 20th. Jeff had gone home to spend time with Will and take him to breakfast with Santa, so a few of my girlfriends had agreed to split time to make sure someone was always with me. I was having a tough day. I had gotten a larger trachea tube put in the day before and I woke up to some bleeding. My good friend Stephanie Anderson was staying with me. Stephanie and a new nurse had continued to talk about my throat. Both thought the bleeding was more than should be occurring. As they were discussing this, two women wandered into my room. I had never seen them before in my life and assumed they were in the wrong room. Nope. They introduced themselves to me and Stephanie. They were from the Baptist church around the corner and a member of our family had-asked them to come. Very kind and sweet, just rough timing as I felt super crappy and was bleeding profusely.

Stephanie worked hard at talking to them and trying to answer all of their questions about me since I could not talk. Then they asked more questions and more questions, and I realized this was not going to be a short visit. They were settling in for a while. I remember feeling very agitated. I just wanted to go to sleep. I was tired and cranky and trying to put on my friendly face, even though I could not actually move any muscles in my face. Finally I decided, I'm the one who is sick here, and if I need to sleep, then by golly I am going to sleep. So I closed my eyes. Poor Stephanie. She tried asking them nicely to leave, mentioning that I was really tired and not feeling great. They did not get the hint, but kept asking questions. More than an hour later they finally decided to go. Stephanie followed them out of the room so she could go to the bathroom. They followed her in there and asked if they could come back in my room to ask me a question about what church I belonged to in Libertyville.

"NO!" Stephanie put her foot down and said, "Carrie is exhausted and needs rest!"

She thanked them again for coming and shared our appreciation (and I was appreciative – just really tired). They indicated they would come back in a few days to visit again. Turns out we never saw those two ladies again Trust me, I did appreciate their prayers! I needed all the prayers I could get.

It was amazing all the prayer groups from across the country I had praying for me. Members of the church where Jeff and I got married back in Lincoln were huge supporters. They sent tons of cards, letters, a cross, and even a prayer shawl for me. You never know when you are going to need prayers and it helped to have so many worldwide!

I loved getting Facebook posts and text messages. Jeff or my friends would read them to me. But the best was the good old US Postal Service mail. Mail was often the highlight of my day. I know I sound like I'm eighty years old right now, but believe me, knowing someone is thinking of you and sending positive thoughts is huge during a recovery process. Snail mail is so rare these days, but in the hospital it was awesome to receive. Since I could not hold cards in my hands let alone open an envelope, whoever was staying the night with me would often open my mail and read me the cards. Many a night I had tears streaming down my cheeks and Jeff or one of my best girl friends would get a Kleenex and wipe the tears off my face. I was touched by all the people who were pulling for me. In a situation like this, you don't realize the power of your network – that web of people you have surrounded yourself with for the past thirty-five years. People I had not talked to in years would come out of nowhere and send me a card, or a note on Facebook, or flowers. The outpouring of love was amazing. Never once during my hospital stay was my room bare. From day one, I had balloons, cards, flowers (once I got out of the ICU), and a few extra fun things that one of our friends from Lincoln sent.

Elizabeth Pruett is a school teacher, so I am guessing these creative genes are instilled in her. One day a big package arrived in the mail. It had a homemade blanket with *Cars* characters on one side and *Planes* characters on the other. It was super cool blanket for Will to use when he came to visit me. She ended up making another blanket for Will when he came to visit Nebraska later. The package also had a jar of Hershey's Kisses labeled "Nurse Bait" with a cute note that all the nurses got a huge kick out of. The box also contained a huge homemade banner with lots of quotes and motivational phrases. We strung it across my entire room and it really brightened my days. I swear it was one of the reasons I got a single room for so long. Later at the rehab hospital, I realized the staff did not want to take down that banner and put it back up in another room. It had taken Jeff a good hour and a full roll of masking tape to get it up on the wall!

December 24, 2013

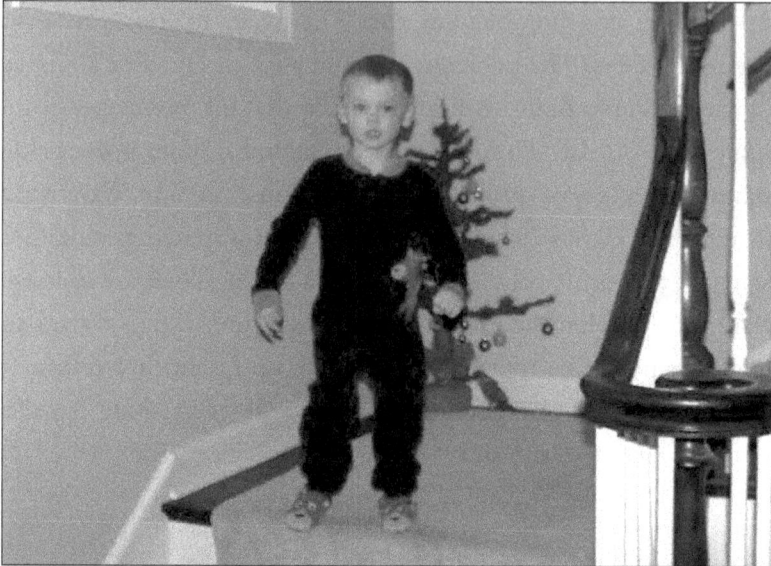

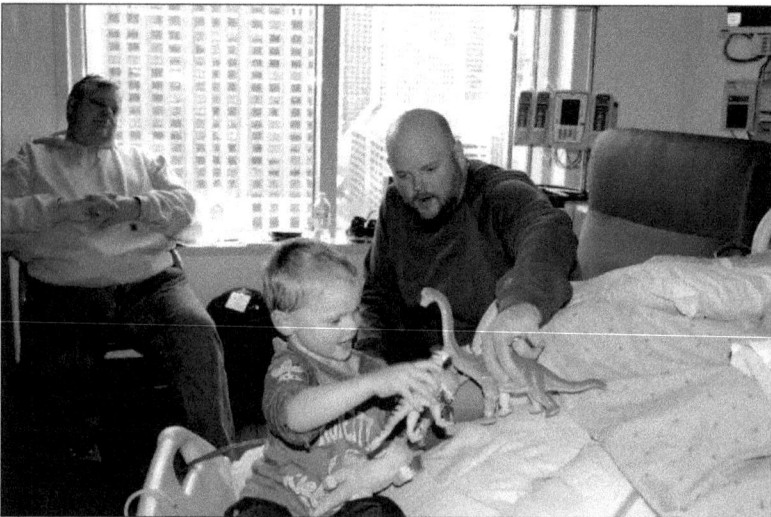

Top: Will on Christmas morning. Bottom: Will playing dinosaurs on Mom's bed with Dad. (Uncle Andy in the background.)

Tue, Dec 24, 2013 at 3:04 P.M., from Jeff's email:

Update for Tuesday, December 24th

Carrie had her fifth and final plasmapheresis treatment early this morning and has had her jugular IV removed. Her neurologist has told us now we're just waiting for the surgery team and respiratory team to clear her for moving to the Rehabilitation Institute of Chicago, or RIC. Once we're cleared by the docs here, we'll work with the RIC doctors on starting rehab there. The doctors have warned us that rehab will very likely be a long process. We're also still trying to figure out the details about weaning off the breathing machine and removing her trach and stomach tubes. She's glad to finally be done with the treatments as they really wipe her out. Now she'll be wiped out by therapy and rehab!

She is feeling somewhat stronger in her shoulders, arms and hands. She's also getting a little feeling back in her legs as we stretch and move her each day.

We wish you all a Merry Christmas and Happy New Year! Carrie and I will be able to watch Will via FaceTime or Skype tonight as he opens some gifts, and then the whole Libertyville crew is going to bring some presents down to the hospital tomorrow. I am sure Will will be all too happy to help mom open her gifts!

Jeff

Christmas Eve – one of my favorite nights of the year. I have so many fond memories of this night. As a child we would go to church at seven and come home to have soup or appetizers for dinner. We would get our comfy PJs on then open all of our presents from my parents. It was a magical evening as the lights twinkled on the tree and presents and wrapping paper were all over the living room. Afterwards, we would head to bed to then wake up to presents from Santa the next morning.

This might have been one of my toughest nights in the hospital. Jeff stayed with me, thankfully, as I could not imagine being alone. But I also felt bad that Jeff was missing Christmas with Will. At three and a half, Christmas is pretty darn exciting, and Jeff was stuck soothing his paralyzed wife in the ICU at Northwestern Memorial Hospital. Not the Christmas anyone dreamed of, but we made the best of the situation.

On Christmas Eve, we Skyped with Will, my parents, and my brother while they opened presents. Will spent a lot of time running up to the iPad and showing us the cool presents from Mimi and Papa and Uncle Andy. They showed us the tree that Will and Jeff had decorated while I laid on the couch watching the first weekend I had gotten really sick. It was hard. My eyes were misty thinking of all the places I would rather be than in a hospital bed.

"Why me?" I prayed that night to God. I remember asking Him to help heal me, to help me walk again, to help me hug my son again. I think I fell asleep a few times praying that night. Then I would wake up and remember where I was and start praying again. It was all I could think to do.

The next morning, we Skyped with Will as he took in all the presents Santa had brought. How wonderful to get to see his expressions, his excitement, his sheer delight. But it also stung. It stung that we were not there in person to hug Will and hear his squeals of joy. It stung that Jeff had to sleep on the chair in my room that would not pull out. It was hard that we missed Santa's visit. My parents and brother were troopers. They packed up Will and some presents for me and came down to the hospital. We were supposed to be visiting Lincoln for Christmas.

"If you wanted us to come to Chicago for Christmas, you could have just asked." Andy said as he walked into my hospital room. He was always the one cracking jokes through this ordeal. He told me everyone else was so serious he had to break the tension with humor at times. I would have expected nothing less from Andy.

Will sat on my bed, which was the best part of my day. He had on his new Nebraska sweatshirt that Andy had given him. It was about three sizes too big, but he loved it. He immediately asked where the presents were. The kid had gotten a bit spoiled with all the presents in the last thirty-six hours.

"Ahhh, we'll work on the spoiling–next year," I thought. "Poor kid deserves anything right now."

Will's whole world had been turned upside down. His mom, his rock, was very sick. He prayed that the doctors would make her better. It was a tough situation, but he was resilient. At the hospital, he would sit on my bed with a pillow behind him facing me while he watched the iPad. I loved watching his expressions—his smirks, scowls, looks of fear, and then smiles. I wanted so badly to reach out and move my hands or even just my fingers to touch his skin. I tried to communicate this to Jeff and to my family, but no one understood that I just wanted to touch Will. I missed him so much.

I wish we would have thought to do something that night for the staff at the hospital. How tough for all of them to be apart from their families as well. No one wants to be at the hospital on Christmas. I hope to never be in a hospital at Christmas time again but if I am – I know now I want to get the staff something.

Will was a huge help in opening my presents. I could not grasp them or tear any of the wrapping. It was the most humbling feeling to be unable to even rip a piece of paper. Will opened them for me. I remember Jeff getting a gift card to go out to dinner. I got jewelry from Jeff and my parents told me they'd bought me the food processor I wanted. I was pumped, but wondered if I would ever be able to use it. What a range of emotions I had all in one day. I was thankful to be alive, to be spending Christmas with my family, but I feared life was never going to go back to the normal I remembered. It was a hard day.

December 28, 2013

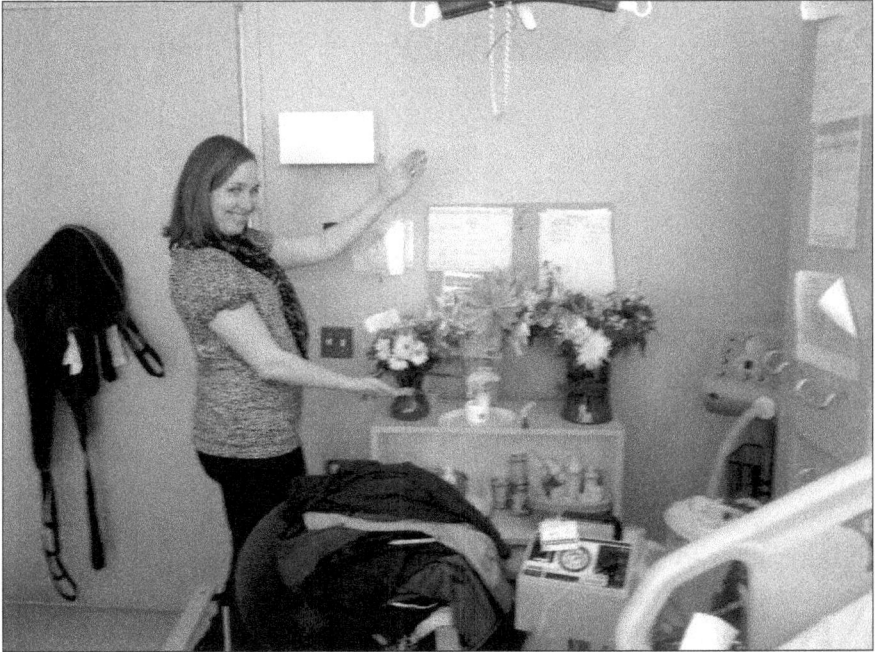

*Carrie's best friend Brooke showing off the flowers in
Carrie's room at RIC.*

Sat, Dec 28, 2013 at 8:59 p.m., from Jeff's email:

Update for Saturday, December 28th

On Thursday, the 26th, Carrie was officially discharged from the ICU. She has been moved to RIC, the Rehab Institute of Chicago, Room 728. She can have flowers, cards, etc. sent to her room now that she is out of acute/critical care.

The adjustment to a new room, new ventilator, and new schedule has been a little rough. She had a full day of evaluation on Friday and today was a rest day. Tomorrow (Sunday) she starts her first full day of rehab — physical, speech, occupational, and others. She has requested that we hold visits until she's more acclimated to the schedule and the work.

We continue to appreciate all of your love and support. She is still showing slow signs of recovery. Prior to today, she could sporadically move different arm muscles. Tonight she showed me she could very slightly move the entire arm from shoulder to fingers. We're thinking positively about the road ahead, but the doctors have told us that we are looking at four to six weeks of inpatient and probably several more months of outpatient therapies.

When they transferred me from the ICU to the Rehabilitation Institute of Chicago (RIC) I was so scared. I still had severe anxiety so any change to my routine was unsettling. How would the ventilator transfer work? How would they move me? What would my new room be like? Would I have a roommate? We had heard that family could not spend the night at RIC, which, if true, terrified me the most. Jeff had been by my side ninety-five percent of this journey thus far. He knew what I needed often before I asked. He calmed me when my heart rate started to climb. He talked to all the doctors and helped communicate to the nurses what I wanted. I was scared shitless that Jeff may not be by my side.

Jeff knew I was nervous. He could tell even though I had no facial expression or movement. He rubbed my arm and told me 100 times it would be okay. I could tell he was nervous as well. He was there when they lifted me on the sheets from the hospital bed to the gurney. They took me down the hallway. I looked around wondering what it looked like. I had been in the ICU for more than two weeks.

We went down an elevator. I remember I was hot. I was always so darn hot. I started to feel suffocated. Jeff told me it was okay. I remember consciously slowing my breathing.

"Deep breath," I told myself.

When we went out the door, wow! The cold burst of air I felt was overwhelming. It had been weeks since I had felt fresh air. It was freezing outside, but I welcomed it. It reminded me I was alive! That cold air was so wonderful. After being so hot all the time in the ICU, the air felt freeing. But in the ambulance, I began to feel hotter and hotter.

"Deep breaths," I told myself.

Jeff rode with me during the transfer. You know what I really hate about transferring via ambulance? They literally wrap like six seatbelts around you and pull them super tight. That's after they wrap you in sheets and blankets. So you are like a mummy all wrapped up, arms at your side. For a person who is already paralyzed, anxiety ridden, and hot – it becomes your worst nightmare. Thank goodness the ambulance ride was literally five minutes from Northwestern Memorial Hospital to RIC (now called the Shirley Ryan AbilityLab).

When we arrived at RIC, the lights were so bright. We got in an elevator, and the attendants pushed the button for the seventh floor. This was the last time I would be off of Floor 7 for almost three months. As a person who likes to get out and socialize, I would have said you were crazy if you'd told me then that I wouldn't leave the seventh floor for three months. Throughout this entire journey it was often a blessing that people did not tell me information or give me the worst-case scenario. That would have definitely sent me into a depressive tailspin. For me, it was all about making progress inch by inch, day by day.

"Most people recover from GBS" was my motto. I was going to be most people.

I remember Andrea the nurse. She was pregnant, and I knew right away she would be a sweetheart. She had that motherly instinct that is great for a nurse. Two women from the respiratory department were with her. One of them was Sonia. She is unforgettable. She loved to talk and tell stories, but had this deep accent, so I only understood about every fourth word. She would stop by often to check on me and my ventilator. She took excellent care of me, which was one of the reasons I eventually was weaned off of the ventilator. She pushed me, but at the beginning, she scared me. I remember early on during my time at RIC, begging Jeff to make her leave. She would take me off of the ventilator when she suctioned me, and I would get so scared. She would talk to Jeff and tell him what we needed to do, and I was not sure if we should trust her. Turns out she knew her stuff!

I came to look forward to hearing Sonia's stories. She had a brother who died skydiving. Her husband had some health problems. I'll never forget the night she was checking on me before she went home. At this point, I was making progress. She latched on to my arm and said, "Sweetie, I pray for you every night." It melted my heart to know she thought about me after she left work. Wow, that left an impression on me.

My room, 728, was bleak. I think it was bigger than the ICU. I got my own room, mostly, I think, because I was on a ventilator. That turned out to be a blessing because family could stay if you had a private room. We had a cot and a pull-out chair so people spending the night had their choice. My friend Brooke set up a schedule so Jeff could go home and sleep or stay at Brooke and Jeff's. That was a huge relief to me that first night and for the next few weeks. I had a safety blanket there of my friends and family. I think it aided in my recovery enormously to constantly have someone there supporting me.

I still could not talk or eat or drink anything. My nerves were re-growing rapidly, which was great, but the pain was excruciating. And I was so damn hot. All the time. I would constantly ask for cold washcloths for my forehead. Then I started asking that they be put on my forearms and then my shins. They felt so good for approximately ten minutes, then I would ask to get them cold again. My friends, parents, and Jeff were pros at letting the faucet run a few minutes to cool the water down, getting the washcloth moist, then wringing it out so the sheets did not get too wet which would make my skin prone to sores.

Like every new patient at the RIC, I had to go through an evaluation day to determine where I was in my recovery and what my rehab plan should be. On Friday, staff from physical therapy (PT) and occupational therapy (OT) came to evaluate me. My speech therapist (ST) was not able to come until Sunday. PT and OT did a series of tests similar to what I had experienced in the ICU.

"Try to squeeze my finger."

"Try to flex your arm and push."

"Try to push your foot down."

In response to every direction, I tried so hard to do what they asked, to will my muscles to move and my nerves to fire, but there was nothing. Those tests were downers, as they reminded me of all I could not do and left me with questions of whether any mobility would come back at all. What if I can never lift my arm again? How will I eat? How will I hug? How will I type? Those tough thoughts were brutal to face, but Jeff was often there to help me handle my down moments and days. I tried really hard to be positive around my friends and other family members. I knew positivity was key, but sometimes I had to let it out. I had to cry and feel sorry for myself and be mad at the situation. Jeff was always there for me, consoling me and telling me it would get better. Other times he would give me the tough love speech which I never wanted to hear. I remember I would get mad but minutes later realize he was right, and I would bounce out of it. I have come to realize that I had to practice resiliency and it became my focus to bounce forward. It was not just about bouncing back – it was about beating this nightmare and showing it who was boss!

During the evaluation, PT measured me so they could get me a wheelchair. That sounded liberating but also frightening. A wheelchair. I had never imagined I would be using one at age thirty-six. And it would be a fancy wheel chair at that. My PT explained that I would have a wheelchair with a sensor so I could drive using my head. I had started to get some movement in my shoulders and could move my head slightly. My PT felt this was enough movement to allow me the chance to drive. Watch out! They took all my measurements to find a wheelchair that would work for me and be comfortable. It would take a few days to find the chair and outfit it with the head sensor. In the meantime, they had a wheel chair in my room I would use for showers and another manual wheelchair that the staff would have to push me in until my custom model arrived.

I must tell you I had amazing therapists. My PT, Patrick, was fabulous. He was a fantastic guy and a great therapist. Patrick is passionate about what he does, and it showed in his therapy sessions with me. He was calm and offered great insight into GBS and how we were going to handle my physical therapy. On our first day together, Patrick explained that with GBS, balanced therapy is essential: push the muscles to remember how to perform certain actions, but never do too much. Overdoing can cause setbacks and we didn't want any of those.

And then there was Zoe, my occupational therapist. She was so loving and comforting. She was great at reading people and situations. She had a gentle touch that helped soothe and reassure me. She was kind and considerate of people's feelings. She told me how excited she was to work with me, to help me regain movement in my hands and arms, and to return to daily living activities.

I felt really good about the therapists I'd met. They seemed exceptional. Little did I understand how much time I would spend with them over the next few months.

Because I just felt crappy, I was not allowing most visitors. But one visitor I did allow was my cousin, Mandy. She was great! She could sense when I wanted to talk and when I needed her to just to be there with me. She and her husband Pete set me up with the Audible App so I could listen to books. I had started using the app in the ICU, but there was a downside: I could not reach out and hit pause if a doctor or nurse came in. It was frustrating when the story would keep playing and I would miss part of the book. It probably didn't help that I had chosen the book *Divergent* which is not the most uplifting book in the world. Awesome book, as I later found out, but in the ICU, I realized it was not the right genre for my mental stability.

Listening to books on Audible was helpful. My vision was still really blurry, so I could only watch TV for a short time before I got a headache. I could not talk or communicate easily so carrying on a conversation was difficult. I remember spelling on my communication board to my good friends, T-E-L-L M-E A S-T-O-R-Y. I just wanted to hear what was going on outside of this hospital room. I was interested in the weather, local events, national news, gossip. My mind was fully functioning and I was intrigued by anything visitors would tell. Once I was no longer heavily medicated, I understood everything people told me. The problem was communicating back. My response was often simple words I could spell on my communication board. My friends often joke it was the quietest I have ever been! For a talkative person, it takes a lot of patience to learn how to listen more!

January 2, 2014

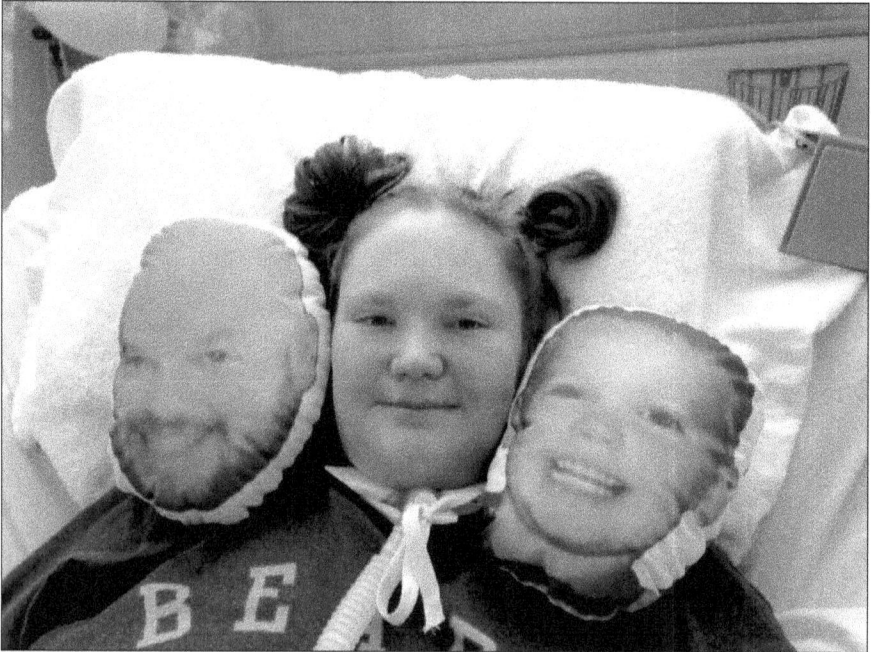

Carrie with Princess Leia buns in her hair, and pillows of her husband and son by her side, courtesy of her friend Patty.

Thu, Jan 2, 2014 at 10:07 a.m., from Jeff's email:

Update for Thursday, January 2nd

Carrie will start her fifth full day of rehab today. We've seen some great results already but of course it's not fast enough for her. She has been able to sit upright in a wheelchair with no issues, along with being able to freely move her arms in a sling contraption that assists against gravity. She's already a pro at driving the electric wheelchair. I credit all those hours of *Mario Kart* and *Need for Speed*!

The doctors, respiratory folks, and speech therapist are thinking that they may be able to modify her breathing tube in the next few days to try some initial speech and swallowing tests.

She also had her first shower on Tuesday. She was absolutely thrilled to have clean hair.

I try to read her your emails every day. She loves to be read your notes of encouragement, love and support, and especially loves to see pictures of her family and friends.

Jeff

The entire time I was in the ICU I was bedridden, and could not get up to take a shower. I've already mentioned how scary bath time was when they turned me what felt like 100 times, my heart rate skyrocketing. A few times, they washed my hair with this powdered shampoo. I was not a huge fan. They would put the powder in and then put a shower cap on my head so that the shampoo could percolate. They removed the cap but never rinsed anything out, so it felt like the powder was just sitting in my hair. And it caused my head to itch like crazy. The kicker was I could not scratch my head since I was paralyzed. And communicating that my head itched was near impossible, so I suffered through it. It also smelled like when I used to get a perm when I was a kid. All in all, not a fun beauty experience!

One of the most exciting things moving to the RIC was that I was going to get a shower. I remember dreaming of the warm water, the cleanliness I would feel. But then fears started to creep in. How would I get out of bed? What would they do about my vent? How would I breathe?

Turns out each room on my floor at RIC had a Hoyer lift. So, on Sunday, the nurses came in and turned me a few times to put a large sling under my back. It was blue mesh and looked like a big blanket with holes in it. The lift control unit was moved towards my bed and lowered, and the nurses hooked the straps of the sling to the lift. They asked if I was ready and I blinked. I was scared shitless. They carefully placed the vent tubes on my lap so they would not get in the way, and started lifting me. It was excruciatingly painful, but I could not scream or tell them to stop. My face wanted to cringe, but since my muscles were paralyzed no one could tell how much pain I was in. Jeff, though, could see it in my eyes. He asked if I was okay. I blinked because I knew that I had to do this, I had to get out of bed. They lowered me onto a special wheelchair that I would use just for showers and eventually for a toilet, but that was a long ways off!

Once I was in the chair, they explained that they would take me off of the vent, and use an oxygen tank and manual pump to give me air during the shower. They removed my hospital gown and taped a bag around my PICC line, a thin tube in my arm that was used to give me medication and to draw blood. They asked if I was ready. I blinked. I could hear the water running. I was so excited to have a real shower after almost three weeks. I was beginning to understand how people on those reality shows feel when they don't shower for weeks. I could swear some animal had made a nest in my hair and that I had a layer of dirt all over my body.

They wheeled me into the shower. A nurse was pumping oxygen into my vent and the Patient Care Technician (PCT) who assisted nurses was in charge of washing me. I had a pillow behind my head to keep me upright. When they took the pillow away so they could wash my hair, it was impossible to keep my head up. My neck would not work. It hit me again; I was very sick and so weak I could not even hold my head up. At that moment a scene from a movie popped in my head. A little boy is explaining that the human head weighs eight pounds! It dawned on me that is a lot, so I cut myself some slack.

The PCT helped hold my head, put shampoo in, and gave me a soothing but forceful head massage trying to untangle my rat's nest of hair. I was always impressed that those PCTs and nurses seemed to have five or six hands when giving a shower, etc. The only bummer of the shower was that the water was not hot. They did everything they could to warm it up, but the shower was not cooperating. Fortunately, maintenance resolved the issue in a few days.

After my shower, they wrapped a towel around my head and a sheet around my body. Then a sheet was placed on top of my bed along with towels, to catch some of the moisture from the sopping wet sling still under me while I sat in the wheelchair. They then brought the lift over and hooked it up. During this time, they had to keep giving me manual breaths from the oxygen tank before reconnecting my vent. While the shower was so refreshing and felt wonderful, the process was exhausting. It felt fabulous though to have a shower! The water running down my body was such a comforting experience after weeks in the ICU.

They reconnected the straps on the sling to the lift. It seemed like I was on a ride at an amusement park, but it wasn't at all amusing, because of the extreme pain in my regenerating nerves. Originally I was taking pain medication every six hours. I finally had to ask the doctors if I could take it more frequently as it just didn't seem to be working. It was changed to every four hours, which helped a great deal. I could always sense when it had been about four hours as my body would start to have a dull ache all over that would progressively get worse.

Once they had me back in my bed and had taken the sling out from under me (a maneuver which involved my oh so favorite log roll), they made sure I was dried off. The worst thing to have in the hospital is a bed sore. Unfortunately, I had arrived at RIC with a bed sore on my tailbone. The nurses and PCTs take bed sores VERY seriously. If you are not familiar with bed sores, they are areas where skin is rubbed raw and a wound opens up. These wounds can turn into very serious infections, so hospital staff watch them very closely to make sure they do not get worse. They made sure to move me every few hours so I was not lying on one specific area too long. My bedsore healed up fairly quickly over the course of the first week or so at RIC, but if I happened to lie on my back too long, my tailbone would start to hurt.

The shower over, it was time to get dressed—another new phenomenon for me. They had asked Jeff to bring gym clothes—loose-fitting, comfortable clothing I could wear to do therapy. Have you ever had your husband pack a suitcase for you? Oh, how I love Jeff, but packing my suitcase was not his forte. He brought a bag to my room, started unpacking my things, and most of the shirts were long-sleeved. I understood that it was ten degrees outside, but apparently he forgot that GBS made me hot all the time. Yeah, I was not so interested in long-sleeved shirts. He did bring a few of my favorite soft comfy shirts and shorts. He also brought workout capris, but I did not want any more clothing than was absolutely necessary.

Another consideration with clothing was using the bathroom. I wore a diaper much of the time. Thankfully, I am not a modest person. Let me forewarn you that if you are modest and have to face a situation like GBS, you will have to throw that modesty out the window. I could feel when I needed to pee and would tell the PCT or nurse I needed to use the bedpan. There was no getting to the bathroom quickly. Using a bedpan is not comfortable at all. They had to log-roll me over, shove that bedpan under me, roll me back over on top of it and hope they positioned it right which occurred about sixty percent of the time. The other forty percent of the time they would roll me back the other way, try to readjust the bedpan, and then roll my body back on top of that hard, cold plastic thing. When your nerves are re-growing and every inch of your body is ultra-sensitive, rolling on a bedpan is one of the most uncomfortable things you can imagine. And how many times a day do we pee? Yeah—bathroom situations were not a favorite topic in my room. So, they would put a diaper on me, negating any need for underwear, then put me in my shorts and a t-shirt. The PCTs and nurses were extremely skilled in dressing me quickly and efficiently. I think they asked me if I wanted to put on a bra. That seemed like it would require extra energy, so I chose to go braless for a good two months. A woman with my bust should never go braless, but at that point I could not have cared less. I was not there to impress anyone. I was there to get better. Looking back, I can see that was one of the reasons all the pictures of me at the RIC are so wonderful! So freshly showered, with my diaper, shorts, t-shirt, and no bra, I was dressed and ready for my day.

Right before the new year, my official wheelchair arrived. I was anxious to get into it and be mobile. A PT was scheduled to teach me how to use it. I was nervous and excited to see if I could drive the wheelchair with my head movements. Before telling you about learning how to drive my new wheelchair, I'll need to explain how therapist assignments worked. I didn't always see my main PT, since I received therapy six days a week and my therapist might have a day off or be seeing other patients. I got to meet and work with almost every PT on the floor, which was great, because each PT came up with different ideas on how to challenge me or push me to the next step. I appreciated that all the therapists were very interested in my progress. Every Monday, all the therapists—physical, occupational, speech, respiratory—and the doctors and nurses discussed my case. They would talk about my progress as well as my challenges and then set their goals for the coming week. It was a pretty cool system that allowed all the therapists to understand and become invested in my case. I am a very goal-oriented person, so each Monday I would ask the therapists what my new goals were for the week and was motivated to blow those out of the water!

It was time to learn to drive. A new PT arrived and asked if I wanted to get up and get in my wheelchair. I blinked with my good eye. (I wonder if I looked like a pirate, blinking with that one eye. Aarghhh...I digress.) Getting in the wheelchair involved using the Hoyer lift. After the shower experience the day before, I knew the lift was going to be painful. As I came to learn over the next few months, many times I had to suffer through pain to continue on the road to recovery. I would just have to bear it. The nurse and PCT helped the PT get the sling under me which involved log rolling again. Still wasn't my favorite thing, but now that my breathing was more stable on the vent and I was used to it, I could handle it a little better.

Before I was moved into the chair, the PT, PCT, and a nurse put me in my socks and sneakers. I thought it was odd at first, but now I think it was a way for me to get in the right mindset for therapy. It was like I was getting ready to go to the gym. They got the sling ready to go then pressed the magic buttons that controlled the Hoyer which lifted me up and over to the chair. The nurse was in charge of the vent tubes to make sure they didn't get caught. The PCT held my legs, and the PT operated the controls. It took a pretty good Hoyer operator to make sure I landed squarely in my wheelchair, and to make sure I was not crooked or sitting uncomfortably. After they got me in the chair, they had to get my vent unattached and put on a cart that could be wheeled next to my wheelchair. Going anywhere was going to take an army—but I was out of my bed! It was such a relief to be up and mobile. Lying in a hospital bed is amazingly horrible for your body. Your muscles lose strength quickly and become tight, diminishing your range of motion.

Once I was safely in my new wheelchair, they buckled my seatbelt. The staff, I would learn, was meticulous about that seatbelt. The chair had two speeds: tortoise and rabbit. The PT clicked the lever to ensure the chair was in tortoise mode, and asked if I was ready to go. I blinked.

Even at tortoise speed it was hard for someone to drive my wheelchair when I was in it. Imagine trying to drive a remote-controlled car while holding on to the side. Plus we had to wheel the ventilator on the cart alongside or right behind me, and sometimes a pole holding the bag connected to my feeding tube came along for the ride. We also had to bring my suction machine. My husband has always made fun of me and the number of bags I always carry. Whether it is going on a trip or just to a friend's house for dinner, I somehow always end up toting several bags, so this was no different. To leave my hospital room required at least two people with me to help roll everything we needed.

We made it into the hallway, and the PT asked if I wanted to drive. The wheelchair had a head array system. I could push with one side of my forehead to make the wheelchair go left, the other side of my head to go right and push my head back to go forward. There was no reverse. Driving sounded fun, but also like a lot of work and I was tired. I was still just not feeling like myself and anything that took a lot of energy seemed overwhelming. I was also nervous and scared.

What if I could not do this?

What if I would be in this wheelchair the rest of my life?

What if my head could not control the head array and I drove into the wall?

I swear sometimes those PTs could read my mind. The PT helping me that day said, "I promise I will not let you crash or run into anything." I hesitated. She asked again, "Would you like to drive?"

So I blinked.

"Was that a yes?" she asked.

I blinked again.

Jeff and the PT both said, "I think that is a yes!"

So they stopped the chair and switched it to P3. (P1 was reverse, P2 allowed the joystick to work, P3 was the head array.)

"Ok, now try to lean your head to the left."

I willed my neck and head to move to the left. I felt like I was pushing so hard, but nothing was happening. Everyone was staring at me.

"Ok lean your head to the left," the PT said again.

I tried to push my head over again, and all of a sudden, the chair started to veer to the left.

"Good!" the PT shouted. "Now stop!"

She pulled the emergency brake on the back of the wheelchair. Now she wanted me to try to the other side. The right was much harder. I could not get the needed pressure. Jeff and the PT tried to adjust the head array—the sides could be pushed closer together or pulled farther apart—so they tried to push in on the right side. I was not as strong on my right-side, which would be the case through my entire recovery. My left side came back more quickly and stronger. To this day, my left foot seems to have more feeling than my right foot.

The PT said that was a good effort for my first time and she drove the rest of the way to the gym.

The gym was a bit intimidating. I have been in plenty of gyms in my day, from basketball courts, to weight rooms, to athletic gyms to work out, but a therapy gym had lots of unique machines and toys. I was not sure what to expect. I could move my left shoulder and blink an eye. What could I do in the gym? They asked if they could put me in the Hoyer lift to get me on the mat. The mat is a table about the size of a queen-sized bed that is lowered or raised based on what the therapist is doing. They put a few foam pieces shaped like cheese wedges on the mat. They told me they were going to lean me on the wedges. I was nervous. As they started lifting me, the pain returned, my body ached, and my face must have shown it. The PT got nervous and was asking me lots of questions.

"Are you okay?

"Should I stop?"

"What hurts?"

They put me back into my wheelchair and took my blood pressure and heart rate, which were both a little elevated. Anytime I was moved, the pain came shooting through my body. But that pain was difficult to describe to nurses, to Jeff, or to anyone.

Through the communication board, I told the PT and Jeff that it was painful to go in the lift, but I would be okay. I said I wanted to try again. So they moved me over, and I sucked it up through the pain. This isn't like paper cut or hangnail pain. This is deep, you want to scream at the top of your lungs pain. Sometimes, I would have to ask the PT to have the nurse bring my pain medication to the gym. I often felt like I was abusing the drugs because I would watch the clock to the precise four-hour mark when I could ask for my pain medication again. I now understand when people talk about how pain management is so important, how if you don't stay on top of the pain, your progress can really be set back. Pain is nasty but it's what I had to endure to recover.

People ask me what was the worst thing that occurred while I was sick. That is really hard to answer because honestly so many things sucked. As I am writing this book, memories start to come back, many of which I'd purposely blocked! One of the worst—especially when I had visitors—was suctioning. When you have a ventilator helping you breathe, your body won't let you clear your throat like a normal person. You cannot go "ughnun" and clear the mucus. In the ICU, they had a built-in suction contraption. The nurse would come in and pump this thing connected to my trach, and it would pull out the mucus. I don't remember a lot about the suctioning in the ICU. I remember it bothered me as it seemed to pull on my trach a bit. (You'll learn later how delicate my throat was.) With the massive bleeding and trauma my trachea went through, I cannot imagine that grabbing the suction pump and jamming it in and out was very helpful.

At RIC, suctioning was even more bothersome. We would have to ring the call button for a nurse. If I needed to be suctioned, a nurse responded pronto. Many times, the act of suctioning keeps a patient from choking to death on their own mucus. Gross, I know. Mucus, saliva, green and yellow crud, it's all disgusting!

Disgusting, and disruptive. After a nurse arrived, a complex process began. Items were readied: oxygen bag, suction machine, suction kit containing a suction catheter and blue gloves (not sure why they were blue, but they always were).

They would then ask me if I was ready to go. See, suctioning involves taking the patient off the ventilator and alternating between drawing up that phlegmy stuff and giving air with a manually pumped oxygen bag. After going through the stress and anxiety of not being able to breathe during my initial transfer from Lake Forest to the downtown Northwestern Memorial Hospital and a few other scares in the ICU, I was not a big fan of going off the ventilator to be suctioned. In fact, it pretty much terrified me early on while at RIC.

Sonia, the chatty respiratory therapist I introduced earlier, was not my best friend at first. Sometimes respiratory therapists would suction me if they happened to be in the room. Sonia would often pause between suctioning me and giving me the oxygen because she wanted to push me to breathe on my own. I did not think this was a fun test at all. I remember I would stare at that oxygen bag and try to will it to come to my mouth. I would start to panic. My heart rate would skyrocket, and Sonia would just be chatting away with Jeff or my mom or, even worse, my dad. If you know Dick, you know how chatty he can be, so pair him up with Sonia and I thought I would never get oxygen again! I would look at Jeff with huge eyes silently screaming, "I need air!" Jeff would nudge Sonia, "Hey – I think she needs some air."

"Oh right, yes," she would say. She would give me a few breaths of oxygen and go on telling her story. I seriously thought I was going to die. It was never that close, but my anxiety made me feel like it was a life or death situation. My heart rate would jump, which isn't surprising. You try having someone stick a tube down your throat while you cannot breathe and then giving you a few breaths with an oxygen bag, and avoid having your heart rate go up.

I know you must be wondering how many times a week I had to go through this horrendous ordeal. It was not a case of weekly, it was a case of daily. Based on where I was in my recovery, it could be anywhere from seven to fifteen times a day. And it was never a fun sight. Some of my friends who witnessed suctioning might be scarred for life!

Suctioning requires a sterile environment because the suction catheter goes down the throat. Once the suction kit is ready, the first step is disconnecting the ventilator and hooking the oxygen bag up to the patient. I would often encourage the person who was with me that day or night to help with the oxygen bag. Jeff, Laura, Brooke, Jennifer, and even my dad became pros at helping provide my breaths between suctions. I must really trust my close friends and family, huh? I had to coach some of them to make sure they did not jam the oxygen bag onto my trachea. My windpipe was delicate, so if the person administering oxygen pushed too hard on the bag, it would hurt something fierce in my throat as if someone had punched me in the larynx. Having my friends and family help provide my breaths was important because let's face it—the nurse only has two hands and I swear it takes at least four to suction properly. The nurse doing the suctioning would use one hand to hold the suction catheter, which was rolled up. The other hand would be on the suction hole. After I would get a few breaths, the oxygen bag would be removed, and the nurse would thread the suction catheter down my throat until I started coughing or they met resistance. Resistance would be mucus. Fluids were really important (through IV at this time) to help prevent mucus plugs, thick clumps of mucus which could make breathing through the vent very difficult. When the catheter met resistance, the nurse would pull the catheter back up while putting a finger on the hole so the machine could do its job and suck the mucus out.

Most of the time the nurse had to repeat this process multiple times to get the mucus out. You can imagine some nurses and respiratory therapists were better at this process than others. Some nurses could do all the steps by themselves and almost were annoyed when I suggested through a five-minute spelling session on the communication board that I wanted Jeff to help. Having him help or my friends help was comforting. I knew they would not withhold oxygen!

After about a week at RIC, I settled into a routine. Brooke, Laura, Jennifer or Jeff would come around dinner time to spend the night with me. They would grab themselves some dinner and sometimes eat in my room. That did not bother me at all. Food did not sound appetizing. I know that sounds odd, especially coming from me. I normally love to eat! I am not sure if it was the ventilator or the pain or the tingling of all my nerves, I was just not hungry. I was also getting about 2000 calories a day through my tube feedings, so it was not like I was starving. While they ate, I would usually watch *Wheel of Fortune*. I felt like I had turned into my father who loves that show. I am not sure why it comforted me to watch. Maybe it was the routine, or maybe it was because it challenged my mind. And frankly, I was concerned it was getting a bit rusty. After dinner, my evening companion would fill me in on his or her day. It was a lot of pressure to come and hang out with me as I could not talk. My company would have to tell me stories. I would often try to ask a question via the question board (a new board that had a list of questions I could point to) to engage in conversation. That usually took so much time that by seven, I was exhausted. These were the times I would get depressed. I missed being able to talk to my friends, to ask questions. I love to ask questions. Then we would sometimes watch TV, and they would massage my arms and legs and put cold towels on my limbs.

My main words and requests to my family and friends were:

T-A-L-K when I wanted them to tell me stories.

M-A-S-S-A-G-E. Though it was painful to be touched in the beginning, as my nerves began to heal, I just loved having my arms, fingers, hands, and legs touched and massaged. It really helped ease the nerve-growing pains. The pressure seemed to dull the tingling. I would pray that my family and friends would volunteer to do this.

H-O-T. I think you get the picture on this one. I've only mentioned it a few times, right? I was still so crazy hot.

W-A-T-E-R (I wish). I kept asking my friends, the doctors, the nurses, and my speech therapists for water. They kept telling me we could not risk it until my throat muscles got stronger. They were right. I did not need to get pneumonia.

T-U-R-N when I wanted them to rotate me in bed to avoid bedsores. Additionally, I would hurt if I was in the same position too long.

January 6, 2014

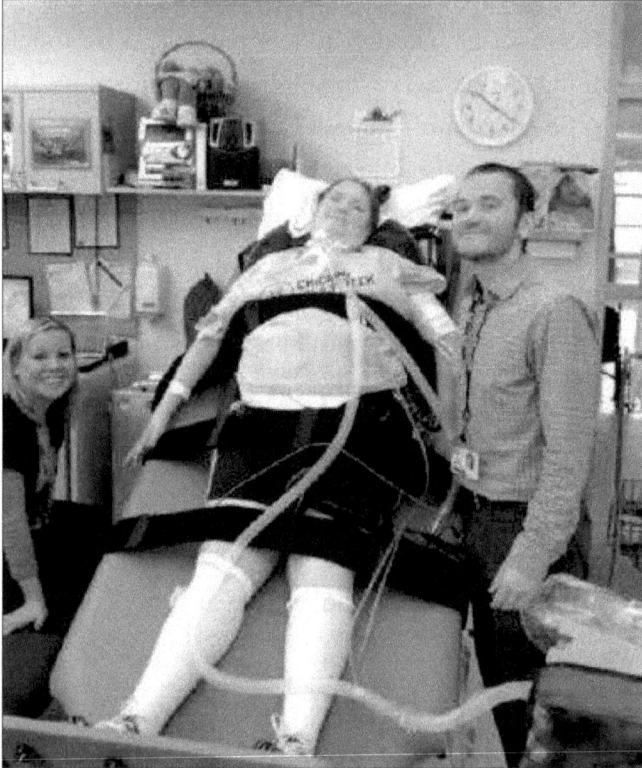

Carrie on the Tilt table with PTs Jill and Patrick.

Mon, Jan 6, 2014 at 5:23 p.m., from Jeff's email:

We spoke with Carrie's doctors this morning and we are very hopeful the ENT people will come tomorrow. We also are hoping to see a neuro-ophthalmologist as Carrie is still struggling with blurry vision - very likely because her facial muscles are not yet back up to strength and her eyes aren't tracking together. Our respiratory folks here are ready to go with their speech tube plan but it has to be approved by the Northwestern Memorial Hospital ENT team.

Today's speech therapy went pretty well, but the music therapy was a no-show. This afternoon we did a combination art and occupational therapy by using a paintbrush with an arm lifter to work on shoulder, elbow and upper arm movement. It went really well, and she may be giving Will a run for his money on the artwork. After OT was PT, and she did almost twenty minutes at forty-five degrees standing up on the tilt table, which is fifteen degrees higher than she sits in bed. She did really really well for basically her first time standing in a month.

She's getting better at rolling her eyes at me when I make bad jokes, so she's definitely feeling more herself lately. Still working hard every day, but all the therapists have agreed she is definitely stronger now than when she came in for first evals on 12/27. Small progress is still progress.

Jeff

I remember doing that first art therapy. I was annoyed I could not lift my arm to just paint a picture. It seemed so silly that my brain could not make my arm lift up. I remember Zoe, my OT, putting my arm in the sling. I remember the art therapist who meant well but didn't like that I was okay with mixing various colors of paint. She wanted me to paint the entire page and frankly I was fine with a little white space, especially when my arm was getting tired. I wasn't trying to get my picture hung in the National Museum of Art. We hung the pictures in my room and a few people asked if Will had painted them for me. I did admit they were my handiwork, and people seemed embarrassed. I would mouth "It's okay." My body is literally like a two- or three-year-old's.

"Day by day, inch by inch," I kept telling myself.

Unless you have to go through it, you don't think about what the body has to endure lying in a hospital bed; how quickly your muscles atrophy and you lose much of the strength you have had most of your life. Physical therapists are all about getting you up and out of that bed and moving. So, the first few PT sessions in late December and early January were literally about getting me up, out of bed, and into my wheelchair. We would head into the gym and they would lift me out of my wheelchair and onto the mat. For at least the first few weeks, my goal was to balance myself in a sitting position on the mat. As I sit here now in my office chair, that seems outlandish and crazy. But my abs and my leg and arm muscles were all extremely weak, and some were still paralyzed. It was a momentous occasion when I could sit on the mat with my hands next to my legs and balance myself holding my head and neck up. I remember being so proud of myself that day. I was making progress. I still had a long way to go, but I actually sat up!

"How about trying the tilt table?" Patrick asked one day. I had seen the table sitting in the hallway but had not seen anyone on it yet. It kind of reminded me of the Frankenstein movies when the monster is strapped onto the table then comes alive! To be frank, I was not so sure of this next step. I had not been upright for over a month. Standing seemed impossible because my legs were still completely paralyzed. But I learned over the course of my GBS journey that you trust those therapists. They know what to push you to try and where to set limits. So I mouthed "yes" to Patrick.

They took me out of my wheelchair in the fun lift. I still say fun sarcastically. Eventually it got easier, but I cannot describe the pain when they moved me and my muscles were tight, my nerves were angry, and I really just wanted to crawl up in a bed and sleep. They laid me on the table and started hooking huge Velcro straps around my lower legs, upper legs, and chest. I started wondering if this was some kind of torture treatment!

My body wasn't used to being upright, so they took my blood pressure often to be sure it didn't drop too quickly, which would cause me to pass out. Then they started tilting the table ten to fifteen degrees at a time towards an upright position. As Jeff wrote, I only got up to forty-five degrees the first time I was on the tilt table. According to Patrick, that was a huge win. After not being upright for more than a month, I managed not to pass out on them! But my back was killing me. Since I could not talk, it was hard to communicate that to Patrick. That first day on the table, Jeff was out taking a work call, so I just pushed through. I filled him in later that day so he could relay to Patrick that my back hurt when I was on the table. Easy fix. The next time, they put a foam roll behind my back to support it! It's amazing how much you miss being able to talk to people and explain what is going on with your body and in your mind!

I mentioned Jeff working. I think it's important to acknowledge how wonderful Jeff's company was through our journey. Jeff's boss allowed him to work from the hospital. Jeff would have his computer propped up on a chair, his phone in his hand listening to a conference call, all while trying to read my lips. I don't know how he did it, but for three months he spent at least four to five days a week downtown with me at the rehab hospital. It was a huge accelerator in my recovery. Jeff would help me during PT, help the nurses move me back to bed, massage my legs at night, whatever I needed. I had support around me almost 24/7 which was so therapeutic during the healing process.

January 7, 2014

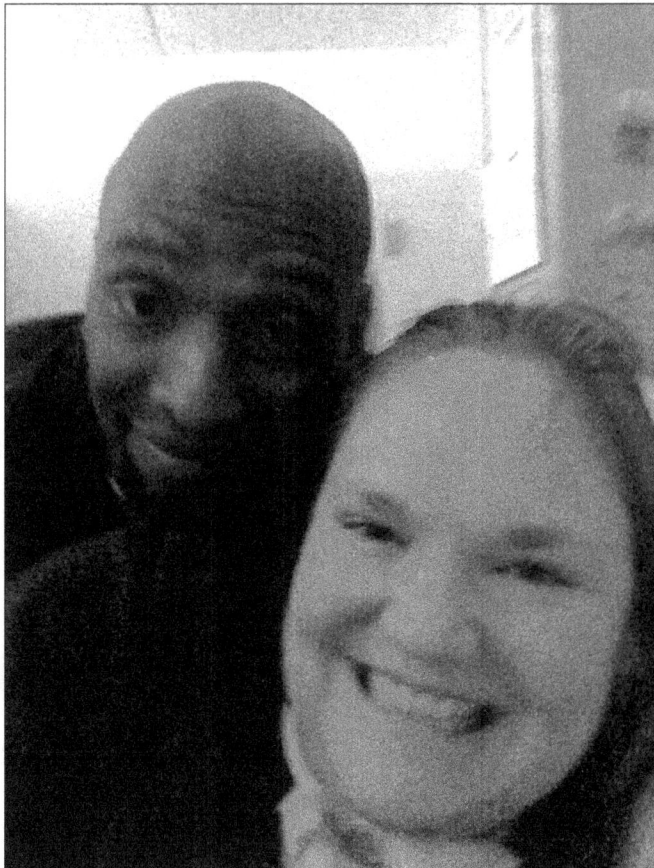

*Carrie and Charles, one of Carrie's favorite
respiratory therapists.*

Tues, Jan 7, 2014 at 2:55 p.m., from Jeff's email:

Update for Tuesday, January 7th

Just a quick update as today we reached a great milestone! The ENT doctors showed up around 12:30 and replaced Carrie's trach tube with the 'Cadillac' of tubes. She rested for a bit with some light leg PT, and then when the speech therapist arrived at two with the respiratory expert, they deflated her trach cuff and she was able to say a few words! Today's progress was to get an initial reading to see what her vent settings needed to be, but she was able to talk for about twenty minutes with me and the therapists, answering questions, clearing her throat and more. Brooke arrived around 2:30 and Carrie surprised her by being able to say hello!

Due to the way the trach and speech works, she still gets tired easily, but a very good sign is that she has not yet needed to go back on supplemental oxygen—doing very well on room air. We are very much looking forward to the next few days of speech therapy as we have a lot more to work on now.

Jeff

I had a love/hate relationship with the Ear, Nose and Throat (ENT) doctor from Northwestern. He came to be one of my biggest supporters, but it would be so frustrating when he was scheduled to come over to RIC, but then he would not make it. If he had any emergencies, he would have to cancel his trip to RIC. If I had been one of those emergencies at NMH, I would want him to do that, but golly it is so disheartening when you are the RIC patient waiting. He was supposed to come and change out my trach and put in a smaller one so they could try leak speech. In leak speech, the ventilator settings are increased, causing some air to leak up to the vocal cords, allowing speech to occur. I was going to be pissed if he did not make it! I was ready to start talking.

Good news! He made it to RIC on January 7th. Getting a trachea tube swapped sounds a bit scary, and you know what? It is! They had to take me off the ventilator, pull the old tube out, and put a new tube in within ten seconds so they could put me back on the machine to breathe. That requires a pretty steady hand. The look on my face before the doctor swapped out the tube must have been something, because he stopped to assure me it would be okay.

Once they got me on a smaller trachea tube, they could try leak speech. Luckily Jeff was there when I said my first few words. I started with "Hello!" It took a lot of effort as I had to talk on the inhale, if I remember correctly. It's the opposite of what you'd think.

Then I said, "This f**king sucks!" and we laughed.

Brooke walked in my room while I was practicing leak speech, so I got to say hello to her. She cried, which made me cry, then my speech therapist started crying. It was a momentous occasion. We were all so happy. I had feared I would never talk again. That would have been very, very difficult for me! They only had me on leak speech for fifteen to twenty minutes that first day as it is very draining on the body and I was exhausted just trying it out. I think I slept for about two hours afterwards!

I forgot to mention that the third thing I said to Jeff was, "I love you." I was so thankful to have him by my side. I think he got a little teary-eyed hearing my voice after a long, scary month!

After a month of communication boards and trying to mouth words, I could finally say whatever came to mind and my mind was blank! I remember wanting to tell a joke to laugh with Jeff. We needed something to lighten the mood after a long December! Doreen, my speech therapist whom I adored, was there with one of the respiratory therapists. I know it was not Sonia, because I think I said, "That Sonia can sure talk!" and everyone laughed.

Doreen was amazing. You can see a pattern here: I had spectacular support at RIC. Doreen had two small girls at home, so she really related to my desire to talk to Will. She was so patient, helping me move along as quickly as possible with talking, eventually drinking water, and eating. Doreen was my cheerleader and I was so happy to have her in my corner.

Water was something I craved. At this point I was not hungry, nor did I want real food. I still felt pretty miserable most days. The smell of food did not bother me because I really don't think I had much of my sense of smell back yet. I don't know if the sense of smell is 'paralyzed' by Guillain-Barré, medically speaking, but food did not appeal to me. Even watching the Food Network on TV didn't make me hungry. Nurses and PCTs would ask me how I could watch that when

I could not eat, but I enjoyed it. I liked thinking about all the things I would eventually eat again.

But water... how I missed water. I am the type of person that carries a water bottle wherever I go. So when I did not drink water from December 9th to the middle of January, it was really tough. I seriously had dreams about water. I woke up and asked the doctor during rounds if today was the day I could have water. Nope. I still had to wait.

I slept a lot while in the hospital. In the ICU, I'd slept on and off most of the day. Sometimes I'd just close my eyes when I had visitors and could not muster the energy to try to communicate any more. I was so tired after therapy at RIC. I remember in January, whenever I would come back from a few hours of therapy, I just wanted to sleep. Getting my body moving again took a lot of energy! My parents and Jeff tried to get me to go to the day room or go on a joy ride in my wheelchair, but I'd be too exhausted. Eventually, I would get to the point where the nurses had to encourage me to go back to my room at night because I liked being out and about. But early on, I could not muster the energy.

I also had gotten into a good nightly routine, which started about nine. I would wait for respiratory to come and do the nightly routine of suctioning me and checking my vent settings. The nurse would then give me my medication which helped me sleep. It was amazing when I started sleeping from 10:30 p.m. to 6:30 a.m., or even later if the nurses and doctors let me!

Soon my wake-up call became the tooth fairy, Adrienne! Adrienne was a hoot. She was in her late fifties or early sixties and worked in the gym helping support the PTs and OTs. In the mornings, she went from room to room to help people who could not brush their teeth. She had an entire system with towels and mouth sponges, and she would give you a hot-towel facial at the end of the teeth brushing.

She thought I was crazy because I always wanted a cold towel on my face in the morning instead of the hot one. I was still so crazy hot, I cannot describe it. It was literally negative ten degrees outside, but I wanted a cold towel! If Jeff was not yet there in the morning, Adrienne would pull up a chair and watch the morning news with me. She took good care of me, was so sweet and always had a smile. Seventh-floor RIC was lucky to have her!

The respiratory therapists were also a hoot. My favorite therapist was Charles, who always worked the night shift. I would try to stay awake waiting for respiratory to come by and do their nightly routine, but often the medication would knock me out before that happened. Charles would come in and be so quiet. He would get everything ready in the dark before he would wake me by gently rubbing my arm. He was like a magician with the suction machine. I swear he had three or even four hands and he could do everything so quickly with little discomfort to me. Some of the other night therapists were not as gentle or as quick with their hands. I know everyone is different and has unique skills, but I wish all the night therapists could have been Charles. I used to ask the nurse, "Who's the respiratory therapist tonight?" I would light up when the answer was Charles.

One of the nurses I really liked, Kristin, always gave me a hard time about having a crush on Charles. She constantly kidded me as she knew he was one of the best. Kristin was a little younger than me and very cool. She had gone through a head injury earlier in her life. She had been hit by a car and had been at RIC for many months. It motivated her to become a nurse at RIC. I think that experience made her a better nurse.

Throughout this journey, I have wondered how to help nurses and doctors comprehend the pain I was experiencing. At times I felt as if no one understood what I was going through. Doctors, nurses, and therapists all may have read about GBS in a textbook, but that pales in comparison to experiencing nerves trying to regrow. Trust me, it's not pleasant.

January 12, 2014

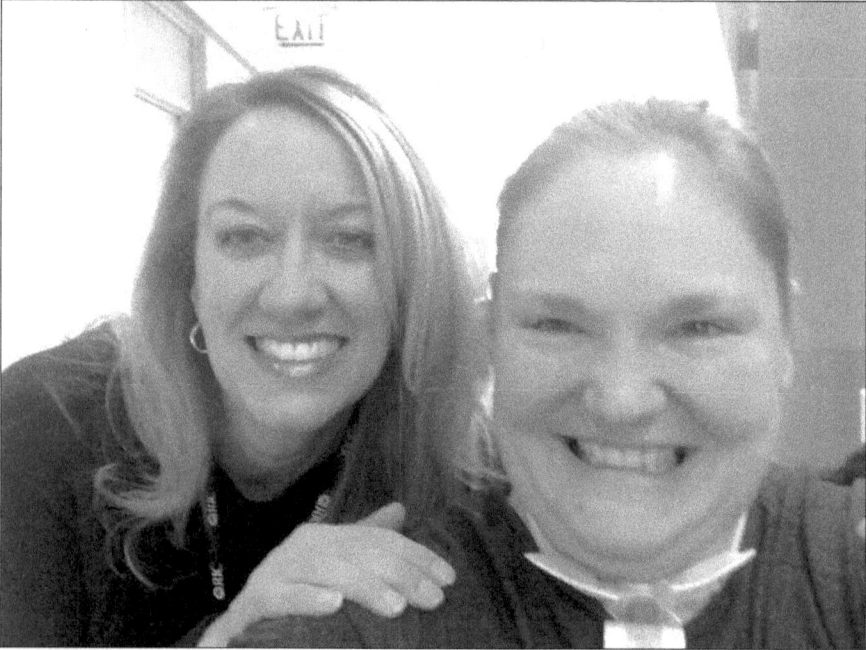

Carrie and her speech therapist, Doreen.

Sun, Jan 12, 2014 at 4:42 p.m., from Jeff's email:

Update for Sunday January 12th -

Thanks to my dad for reminding me it's not actually December anymore.

Carrie had a great week of therapy. The speech has been up and down this week as there's been some discomfort and tiredness with the different trachea adjustments. She is working hard though and was able to swallow a few spoons of water so is very hopeful to continue that and get back to being able to drink and eat. Will came to visit today, and she loved being able to talk to him finally. We also had a visit from a good friend who went through his own bout of Guillain-Barré earlier this year and had lots of great advice and information. Carrie says she feels very motivated to keep getting better. Looking forward to a new week of therapy and improvements.

Jeff

Water. How sweet the taste! My speech therapist started working with me to get ready for a swallow study that was coming in a few days. Leading up to it, they gave me small amounts of liquids and food to see if the more than thirty muscles in my throat were strong enough after paralysis to be able to swallow food correctly. If those muscles had not strengthened, then food and liquids might go down the wrong pipe into my trachea, end up in my lungs, and cause pneumonia. So, the doctors and speech therapists took reintroducing food and liquids very seriously.

Accordingly, Doreen and the other speech therapists worked with me on exercises to strengthen my throat muscles. I also adored my speech therapist, Kyra, who loved the Cubs baseball team as much I do. It was fun to share important things in my life with my speech therapists. They wanted me to talk and communicate as much as I could. I had to put my tongue on the roof of my mouth then sweep it to the back of my throat to mimic swallowing and other not-so-fun exercises. I would do these when I was lying in bed watching TV. Jeff was really good at reminding me to do them so I could drink water!

Doreen started with a few drops of water on a sponge. I carefully slurped up those water droplets then carefully swallowed them. It was heaven: The coolness of the water, the wetness running down my throat! I cannot express the joy. My friend Laura told me that my eyes sparkled when they gave me those sponge water drops. I would suck on the sponge to get the water out of it. I would ask them to go get ice water if the water became warm. I wanted it as cold as I could get it when they dunked that sponge. It also helped mentally with the hotness. There is nothing worse than being hot and not being able to drink water!

That first day, after Doreen administered the sponge, she threw it in the trash so I could not keep drinking from it. The next day, though, she left the sponge and told Jeff he could give me small amounts of water. Jeff and my friends maybe soaked the sponge in the water a little longer in the water cup for me than Doreen had prescribed. The good news, though, was that I was tolerating it! I could feel the water going down the right pipe.

A few times when Jeff or my friends gave me water I could tell it went down the wrong pipe and I would try to cough it up. I was not quite strong enough to cough fully, so I would tell them I needed to stop with the water sponge for a while. As glad and encouraged as I was to be making progress in other areas of therapy, my mood improved even more once I started to get a little water. I had been desperate for the cold, wet, and yummy taste of water!

That weekend, Kent and Ann Seacrest, friends from Lincoln, came to visit me. Kent had battled GBS six months earlier. Kent is about twenty years older than me. We had gotten to know each other through my previous job in Lincoln working on a land development project for our family business. His visit was huge in my recovery! It was so helpful to talk to someone who had suffered this syndrome. It was so reassuring to be able to ask him if a certain feeling or emotion was normal, to compare notes on medications, and to hear of his recovery.

Kent and Ann came to visit on Saturday. I was actually on leak speech, so I could talk to Kent a little bit and Jeff could ask questions, too. Kent told us his entire story, how the GBS came on and how it felt as the paralysis spread. Kent was lucky that his paralysis slowed and did not go above his arms, so he didn't have to go on a ventilator. Kent said he did not regret getting GBS.

"How could he say that?" I recall thinking to myself. This is miserable, and I just want it to be over!"

He told me I'd understand when I was through the journey. He was right. Kent also said that since he had recovered from GBS, he has imposed a three-month rule on how he reacts to life. If he is stressed or worried about something, he says to himself, "Is this going to matter in three months?" He told me all about his rehab and what types of machines they used to help him walk again. He said that he still had numbness in his feet, which really flared up when he was tired or had walked a lot.

Ann was so sweet and spent some time talking to Jeff about how to navigate GBS as a spouse, giving him good information and some tips on coping mechanisms. She also shared some meditation and breathing exercises with us. I had never focused on breathing so much in my life! The tactics Kent and Ann shared helped immensely, not only because they were concrete, specific actions Jeff and I could take, but also because they carried the credibility that comes from first-hand experience.

One of the best pieces of advice Kent gave me was about how to handle the painful and stressful moments. Kent talked about how he hated to be turned (that made two of us!), so he would close his eyes and work on a story. He made up magnificent stories in his head over the few months—so good he should write them down! He said this coping mechanism helped him focus on something positive instead of the pain. I used this story-making concept multiple times while I was in the hospital and it worked well. Ken's insightful tips and tricks helped me persevere.

Kent encouraged me to ask the doctor about a medication called Neurontin (Gabapentin). It turned out to be a life-saver as it cut down the nerve pain I was experiencing. I continued to take the medication during my outpatient therapy as the nerves in my feet continued to grow. It helps calm that pins and needles feeling that never seems to go away.

Kent and Ann came back to see me on Sunday. My friend Jennifer Becker was with me that morning and she, too, benefited from what they had to say. It was reassuring to all of us to see that there can be a happy ending after GBS. Kent and Ann gave us a priceless gift: hope that I would eat, drink, walk, and talk again.

January 16, 2014

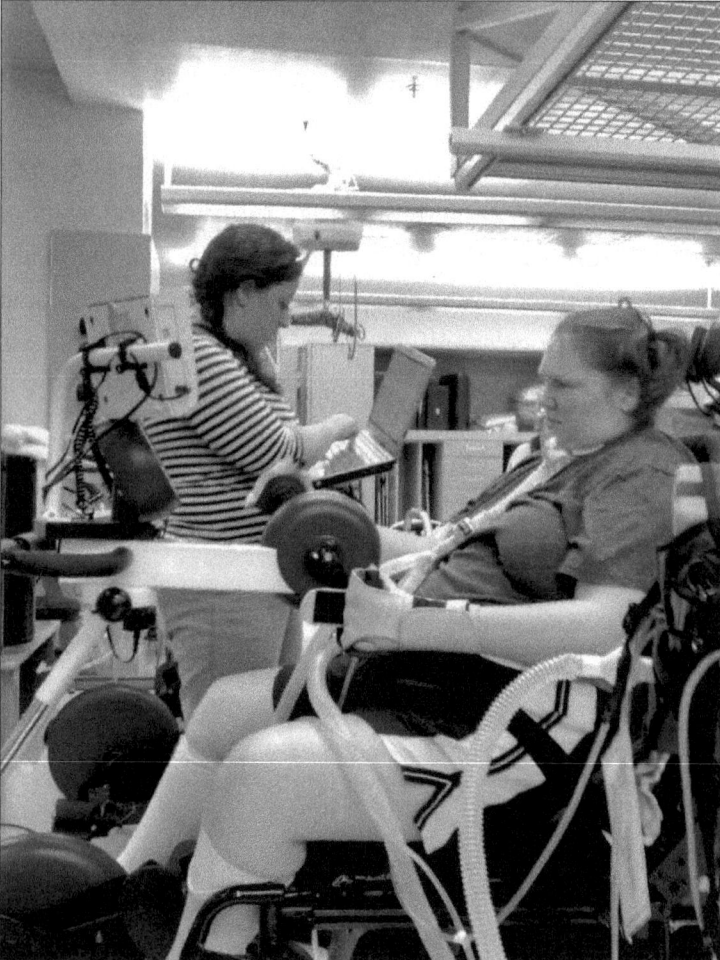

Carrie on the bike with OT Jessica.

Thu, Jan 16, 2014 at 10:27 a.m., from Jeff's email:

Carrie has had a really good couple of days. She's really been focusing on her breathing as respiratory has been lowering her settings while on the ventilator, and making her breathe on her own during suctioning. They've also lowered the support she's getting while on leak speech therapy. They want her to try being on leak speech more and more to build up that strength. Yesterday she was on for almost two and half hours. She also started a new medication called Neurontin to help with the random nerve pain and sensations she's been experiencing. Her nurses mentioned it was odd she wasn't on it before, almost everyone else on her floor already takes it.

PT and OT have been great the last few days as well. She was able to use a spoon attached to a wrist brace to pick up beads and bring them to her mouth to practice eating, and in PT the other day she was able to sit up by herself unassisted for five minutes, rest, and then another three minutes.

The swallow test she was so excited about this week has been pushed back to next week, so she was a little bummed about that. She is doing all of her speech exercises multiple times a day, and practicing with the ice chips and sponge water swallows. She is just ready to chug water as soon as the docs will let her.

Jeff

Weaning off a ventilator is extremely tough. For almost a month a machine had been breathing for me because I was paralyzed. As I started to regain some of those muscles and nerves, I was amazed at how much strength I'd lost. Breathing takes a lot of energy, but I was determined to get rid of the ventilator. Yes, it was keeping me breathing, but it made everything difficult. Leaving my room took at least three people: one to hold the vent, and two to get me in the lift and over to my wheelchair. In a way, the ventilator was a deterrent to me getting better!

So Sonia, the respiratory therapist, began to challenge me. She had faith I could breathe on my own. She stopped giving me oxygen during suctioning. It was scary at first, and I cried to Jeff that I could not do it! But over time, it got easier, and I reminded my brain that we could do this. The mental game was as tough as the physical effort it took to breathe again on my own. Leak speech was also very tiring because I had to produce air to talk and to breathe. Early on, I would fall fast asleep as soon as they took me off of leak speech because I was so worn out. Day by day though, it got easier and easier.

Zoe, my occupational therapist, wanted me to practice using a spoon so I would be ready when I could eat food again. I cannot express how frustrating it is to try to reteach your muscles how to lift a spoon to your mouth. Things we take for granted each day were so difficult to relearn. I practiced with a bowl of beads. I had a splint-like thing on my wrist to help support my hand. I would dip the spoon into the bowl and will a few of those beads to jump onto the spoon. I prayed to God that I could then lift the spoon without spilling a bead and get it close to my mouth. I know we lost at least three beads when they rolled off the spoon and under a cabinet. I tried to throw another handful into my mouth, like I was doing some trick. Zoe said that did not count!

I am so thankful to have had some exceptional therapists helping me progress as quickly as possible. They were always thinking ahead to what was next for me, balancing the need to push me as far as possible while respecting the possibility that going too far to fast could trigger a setback.

January 19, 2014

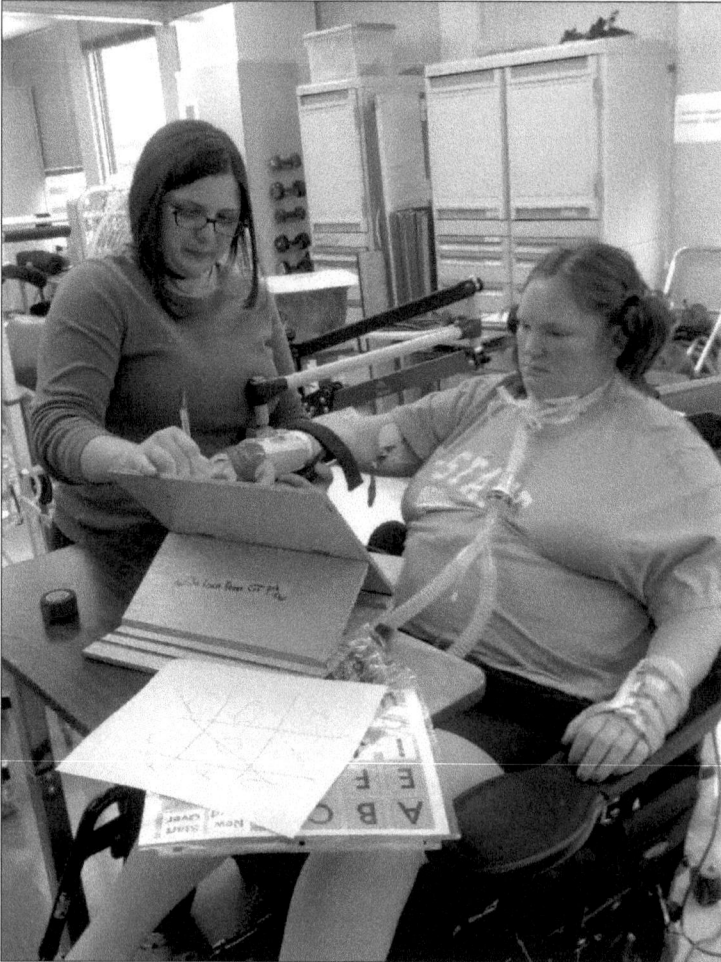

Carrie working on occupational therapy with Zoe.

Sun, Jan 19, 2014 at 7:36 p.m., from **Jeff's email**:

Update for Sunday, January 19th

Everyone on this email already knows, but Carrie is an absolute rock star. I believe the term bandied about today by the therapists was 'badass'. Friday morning she had her first swallow of real food since being in Lake Forest Dec. 9th-12th. She managed five bites of applesauce with no issues at all. She also convinced the speech therapist to let her try a few sips of water out of a straw.

Yesterday (Saturday) was a big day—she had her trach cuff down allowing speech from 10:30 a.m.-4:00 p.m., took a two-hour break and was back at it from 6:00 -9:00 p.m. It may have helped that several of her girlfriends came to see her and she had a lot of stories to tell them.

Today (Sunday) she had another speech therapy and was able to swallow seven bites of applesauce along with several swallows of some thickened orange juice. The plan for tomorrow is to try a soft solid— a graham cracker or similar—to continue to test her reflex. If all goes well, the official barium swallow test is on for Thursday. Her cuff was also down today from 10:00 a.m.-6:30p.m. Eight and a half straight hours with no break. The respiratory therapists have told us she is checking all the boxes to get off the vent, and she's very happy to hear that.

Carrie is also making great strides on the OT/PT front. Today she showed off by waving to Will when he came to visit. She is able to pick up her entire left forearm and wave her hand now. Two weeks ago she could barely move her shoulders. She's doing her jobs—working on therapies and resting—as best she can every day.

She is looking forward to seeing her dad. He flies in this Tuesday through Saturday so I'll be able to get into work a bit more. Will heads out on a Midwest road trip tomorrow, first to Kansas with my folks for a few days, then up to Lincoln to visit the Campbell clan and possibly a new cousin, depending when she decides to arrive.

Jeff

On Saturday, January 18th, my good friend Patty came in from Michigan. Patty is one of the members of my BACH tribe. We have been friends since our sorority days at Purdue. My close friend, Stephanie (we call her Shipley, her maiden name), also a Tri-delta sister, drove up from northwest Indiana. We had a girls' day! They sent Jeff home to relax and play with Will while they entertained me. Stephanie became my nail stylist while I was in the hospital. Right before I got sick, I got a no-chip manicure at my favorite nail salon. Turns out that when you are lying in a hospital bed and cannot move, your nails remain very pretty! My therapists would comment on how nice my nails looked, and ask who did them. After more than a month, the new growth on my nails meant that they were about half painted and half bare. Stephanie volunteered to soak my nails and try to remove the no-chip polish. She succeeded, then repainted my nails. I then got to tell my therapists that Stephanie was the nail tech who made my nails look so good!

BACH tribe members Brooke and Laura joined us that night, and the girls had a bottle of wine and some pizza. My nurse that evening (whom I will refrain from naming so she doesn't get into trouble), pretended not to see the wine and provided some plastic cups. She understood that a little girls' party was important to me and my friends. Even though I could not eat any pizza or have any wine, I was hanging out with my girlfriends. It was great motivation for being on leak speech almost all day. I basically doubled the longest I had been on leak speech yet. I had a lot to say!

I was full of stories, gossip, and information that had been stuck inside my head for over a month. It was such a delight that we could start to laugh about the experiences. Like the communication board and my dad holding it backwards.

I also filled them in on the only therapist that I didn't enjoy working with: the psychologist. Brooke got to help tell that story, as she was with me when it happened. The psychologist meant well, but our personalities just didn't meld. The first time we met was after Christmas and I felt awful! The psychologist was more than an hour late to my appointment. I was enjoying a nap with *Wheel of Fortune* on in the background when she arrived. I couldn't talk at this point, so visitors and therapists had been using the communication board and lip reading. The psychologist asked me question after question. And we are not talking one-word-answer questions. No. It was more like "Tell me what you are feeling and how you are expressing your feelings?" And on and on. She refused to use the communication board. She swore she was a great lip reader. So, after every question, I would start to slowly mouth my response. She'd make me stop and tell me to start over. Because Brooke (unlike the psychologist) could actually read my lips, she would try to interject and paraphrase what I was mouthing. After about six cycles of my starting to slowly mouth a reply to a question, the psychologist telling me to stop, and Brooke trying to summarize, the psychologist said the worst thing anyone said to me during my stay at the hospital: "Caroline (after we had told her to call me Carrie), I would appreciate it if you could articulate your words better!"

I was livid. I shut down and stopped trying to answer her questions. I didn't appreciate her saying this to a person who a few short weeks ago was completely paralyzed, unable to move, unable to speak, and who was now working incredibly hard to regain her muscles to try to articulate her words better.

Brooke knew I was pissed. She calmly told the psychologist I was tired and maybe we could continue tomorrow. I think the psychologist realized she had been rude because she tried to backtrack. When she finally decided to leave, she said she looked forward to our next session. She said that I would grow to like her, quoting her mother, who once told her that she "grew on people like mold grew on aged cheese." That was enough for me. I shut my eyes and pretended to fall asleep. (That was one good escape mechanism I wish I could use in everyday life!)

Food! We started with applesauce because its thickness makes it easy to test the swallow reflex. It went well, so I got a few more bites. I was still not very hungry. I was sick of the liquid diet stuff they pumped through my gastro-tube. It had an awful aftertaste and I seemed to burp it up quite often. The speech therapists had been asking me what I couldn't wait to eat. I was anxious for some McDonald's French fries. I love French fries. And yes, I know how bad they are for you. Come on though, who looks forward to a bite of broccoli?

After the applesauce, Doreen asked if I wanted to try to sip water through a straw. YES, I did! We were pretty confident I would not have the strength yet, but she said we could give it a shot. Doreen had been tipping a regular cup back and having me sip the water that way. I could not hold onto the cup myself or lift it to my mouth, so I needed her assistance. A straw would be much easier.

Doreen came back with the ice-cold water and a straw. She instructed me to sip slowly and carefully. I remember taking a deep breath and then sipping with all my might because I did not think it would work. Bam! Water exploded in my mouth! The look on my face must have been priceless. Doreen ran over to my bed asking if I was okay. I carefully downed the water with a hard swallow and she grinned from ear to ear! It worked! It must have been all that practice I'd had with drinks on the beach over the years! Doreen and I were ecstatic as this opened up a whole new world. If I passed my swallow test later in the week we could set up a drinking system in my room and I could drink water whenever I wanted. I felt like a kid on Christmas! The anticipation of this swallow test was killing me!

Lift up your arm right now. No, I'm serious… lift it up. Seems simple, right? I was ecstatic when I could lift my arm and wave. It was a step-by-step process. One day, slowly but surely, my fingers started moving again. Then I could lift my wrists slightly up and down. Movement! When Will came to visit me on that Sunday and I could lift my arm up and wave to him, I cried! He got a huge smile on his face and said, "Mommy is getting better!"

The next step was to put that arm around Mr. Will and hug him tightly! I wanted so badly to snap my fingers and be healed and walk out of that hospital with my little boy. I so looked forward to all of his visits and loved hearing his stories and seeing his happy face. He would bring me drawings to put on my wall, which made me smile even when he couldn't be there with me.

I also started to have initial muscle response in my hips, quads, hamstrings, and glutes. Those muscles had been paralyzed for more than a month. My physical therapists would test those muscles every few days, and on January 17th, we had response! This was super exciting! My journey to walk again was underway. Such positive news was a huge motivation, an indispensable boost to my hope. It was concrete evidence that I was getting better. I was surrounded on the seventh floor of RIC by many people who had spinal cord injuries, and, in some cases, they were never going to get better. They were not going to get out of their wheelchairs. That was hard for me to think about and to watch. I will give all of my RIC buddies real credit, though—they all cheered me on. I think I represented hope to them that they could recover. They watched me go from being completely paralyzed and driving a wheelchair with my forehead, to getting movement back, day by day.

I was still using the tilt table at this point. I went forty minutes at seventy degrees with no blood pressure issues. As I've said earlier, it's hard to understand how quickly muscles atrophy when the body is immobilized on a bed or in a wheelchair. Standing and putting pressure on legs that weren't functioning was unexpectedly strenuous. I remember one particular tilt table experience when they tried to go to eighty degrees and I made a very angry face. They quickly took me back to seventy degrees and I had to spell out on the board that my quads were on fire. The positioning set off anger in those muscles, but Patrick was quick to point out that this was an awesome sign. Those muscles were firing! You don't usually think of celebrating pain, but I took any celebration I could!

January 23, 2014

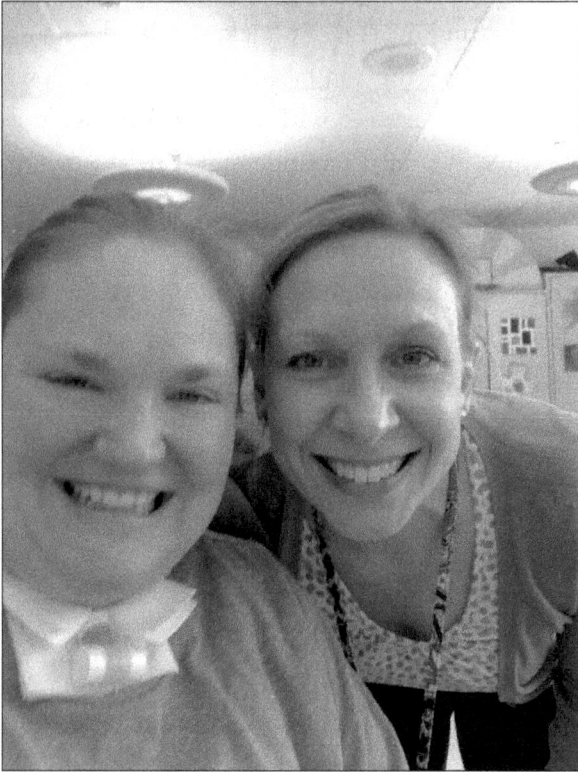

Carrie with Speech Therapist, Kyra.

Thu, Jan 23, 2014 at 6:51 p.m., from Jeff's email:

Update for Thursday, January 23rd

Carrie has made some more great progress this week. I spent Tuesday night and Wednesday at home and in the office, catching up on a lot. Dick has been here this week to stay with Carrie and it has been such a blessing.

When I arrived at RIC this morning, she showed off her new skill of wiggling her thighs and kneecaps at me. So great to see lower body muscles coming alive! She's starting to have less numbness and more pins and needles feelings in her legs as well—positive and negatives there.

The big news for today was the swallow test. The doctors and therapists kept saying it wasn't a pass/fail test, but we feel like she passed because she can officially start drinking sips of water through a straw, and will start working on eating more applesauce, pudding, yogurt, etc. Softer solids will be a work in progress as well. Of the fifteen to sixteen swallows that were recorded, only one tiny bit of liquid went down her trach. She's very excited to be able to drink water!

The rest of today she worked very hard on her therapies and is relaxing now. Hoping for another good night of sleep.

Jeff

Having my dad at the hospital was always a good time. He was such an advocate for me, and always wanting to help. He struck up a conversation with every person who came in my room. Sometimes this annoyed me because I just wanted that person (nurse, PCT, therapist) to help me, but they were all very kind and wanted to answer my dad's questions. Dad even gave Jeff and my friends a few nights off and stayed at the hospital with me. There are not many thirty-six-year-old women who can say they have had a sleepover with their dad!

My dad wanted to help them get me in my wheelchair. As you know by now, this took multiple people. In my mind, the most important role was the person holding my feet up. I am not sure if it was because my nerves were re-growing in my feet, or my muscles were so tight from being laid up in bed and a wheelchair, but when I was hoisted up in that lift, I had to have someone hold the bottom of my legs (under my calves) at a very specific angle to avoid severe shooting pains. Jeff was usually the designated leg holder. It would stress me out if the leg holder had not done it before. The pain was ridiculous when the legs were not at the right angle. It took a few tries for me to train Dad on the correct positioning and holding of the legs, but he was a trooper and took all of my yelling and whiney comments in stride.

One day, Patrick brought in a new face: Jill, a student who was working with him. To be candid, during the first few sessions, I didn't care for Jill. She was stiff and all about business. She didn't seem to care about me or my situation. I did not feel safe with her. Like other PTs, she would take me to the gym, get me out of my wheelchair, and onto the mat, which was about a foot from the floor. She'd then put the foam wedges behind my back. Next, she'd slowly pull me away from the wedges into a full seated position. Because my abdominal muscles were paralyzed, I couldn't sit up. Once the ab nerves started firing, it was possible to use those muscles (barely). I was amazed at how quickly I'd lost core strength. I once took for granted that my body and all its systems—muscle, nerve, and respiratory, most notably—worked together so that I could do mundane activities such as sitting on the edge of a bed. Just that everyday sort of action uses an amazing number of muscles.

That's why physical therapists had to work hard just to get me to sit up on the mat. They lightly held me, forcing my muscles to kick in to keep me upright. It was terrifying. I felt like complete crap. I couldn't move my legs. I felt there was nothing supporting me. That's why Jill was not my best buddy initially. After getting me seated, she would barely hold me! I was scared to death that she would forget I was there, let go, and let me tumble to the floor. I was still on the ventilator making all of this ten times more complicated. I couldn't talk. I couldn't tell Jill how scared I was. But Jill and I did become buddies. I swear it took longer because I couldn't talk. It's amazing how much easier it is to make friends when you can talk, ask questions, and give answers.

After I finally conquered sitting up unassisted, using my ab muscles to hold me steady, the PTs would time me. They would have me try to lift my body off the wedges up to the sitting position. Without leg muscles or full arm strength, that was hard to do. They would push me side-to-side and front-and-back while I was in the upright position. This worked on my ab strength. On January 19th, I sat up for thirty minutes! I remember how proud I was. I celebrated those successes and I think those celebrations fueled my recovery. There was a sign in the PT room that said, "Mile by mile it's hard, inch by inch it's a cinch!" It's a cheesy sentiment for sure, but I couldn't agree more. The type of recovery I was dealing with required that mindset.

The gym had a bike that I could cycle with either my arms or my legs. The PTs would push my wheelchair right up to the machine and strap my legs in the stirrups. The cool thing was that the bike cycled for me, or I could take over cycling if I had the strength. It was good to get on the bike because it got my legs moving and stretched them out, reminding those muscles how to fire. The first time I rode the bike in early January, I had no leg movement at all, so they set the bike to do the majority of the pedaling. I remember concentrating really hard on pushing my legs and the PT was astounded that the controls showed I had taken over some of the cycling. It was a positive sign that my muscles were firing! We were not sure if it was a fluke or the real thing, so a few days later they re-tested my leg muscles and sure enough there were signs of the paralysis receding and my muscles coming back to life! Whenever Jeff returned after being gone a few days, I loved showing him my new tricks. That was a big one! Who doesn't like to show off that their kneecaps are moving?

The SWALLOW TEST. It was a big, big day. Everyone was pumped. My dad was there asking Doreen lots of questions. I had practiced the previous days eating applesauce and graham crackers and drinking water. I was so excited knowing I was on the verge of getting the clearance to drink water without a therapist with me, or Jeff or my friends sneaking it to me with the sponge!

The test was scheduled for 11:00 a.m., but the doctor's schedule pushed it back, so I had to have another stupid tube feeding. I was praying that day it would be my last tube feeding. "Eating" a liquid diet is as fun as it sounds. Nasty!

I was getting more and more nervous about the test by the minute. What would happen if I didn't pass? I was ready to have real food and a glass of water! Eventually, they took me to a small room on a lower floor for the test. I had to drink barium since the test used an X-ray system to detect how I swallowed. The staff filed into the room wearing heavy aprons. I was on one side of the room with my speech therapist Doreen. On the other side, behind a screen, were my dad, Jeff, Kyra (the other ST), the doctor, and the X-ray technician.

The test started with thick liquids, then applesauce, then graham crackers, and then water. I thought it went awesomely. Doreen had no reaction, which I am sure is required of an ST during such a test. We finished then she asked the doctor if I should try swallowing a pill. He said no.

No? I began to worry that I'd failed.

Doreen allowed everyone to come over to our side of the screen. She replayed the video of my test for us to watch. Of the fifteen tests, all but one were perfect. The thick liquid: great. The apple sauce: successful. The graham cracker: stellar. The water to wash down the graham cracker: slight problem. Doreen replayed that portion of the test on the video like seven times, and I swear I could not see the tiny droplet of water that went down the wrong pipe. But the doctor saw it. It was minuscule, and, in my very unqualified opinion, a non-issue. The doctor said I could start eating thickened liquids and pureed foods, but no water until I practiced a week longer.

WHAT???? I was heartbroken. No water today?

We got back to the room and I asked Doreen if I could drink water if Jeff was around.

"You should only be drinking water with a speech therapist," Doreen said. Then she winked.

Doreen left and I told Jeff about the wink. He didn't believe me. I lost it with him. I asked him to go get me a glass of water and a straw. He made the smart decision and did it. So, despite what the doctor ordered, I drank water that day through the straw (when the nurses and doctors were not around) and I was fine! In my mind I was ready, and that stupid little drop of water that went down my throat incorrectly? Forget about it!

January 26, 2014

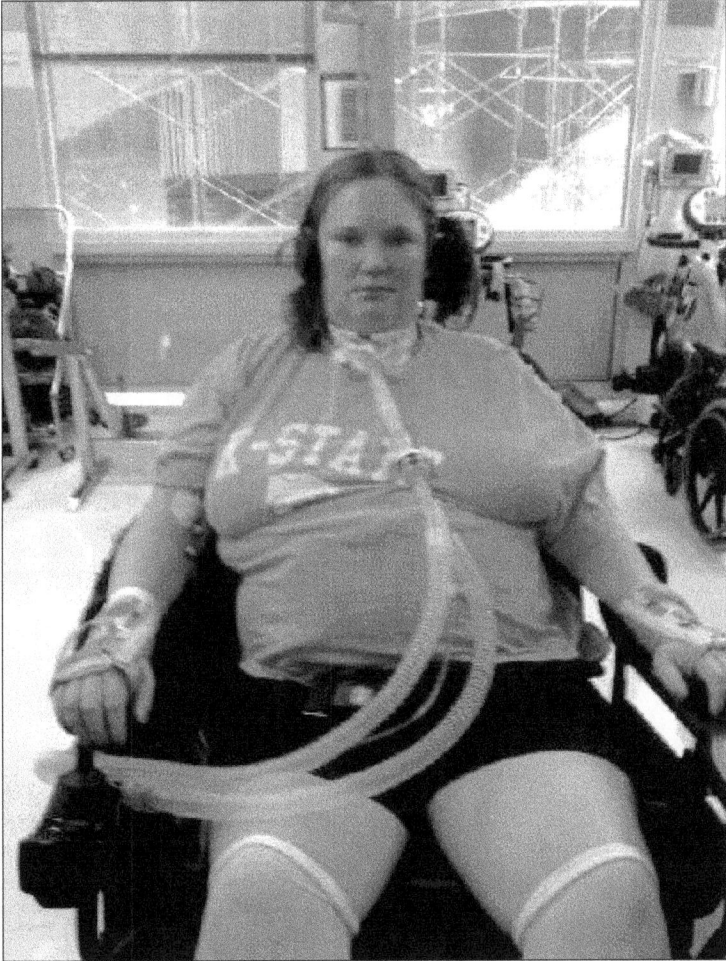

Carrie in her wheelchair with all of her vent cords.

Sun, Jan 26, 2014 at 2:09p.m., from Jeff's email:

Update for Sunday, January 26th

Carrie has very much been enjoying eating—all pureed foods thus far but she's definitely liking it better than the tube feedings. She's craving McDonalds' French fries so we'll have to see when those get the go-ahead! She's working hard on her therapy as well, getting more and more of that lower-body strength back. Her PTs are discussing how they want to start progressing forward from the tilt table, sounds like we have several options to work with.

Jeff

Pureed food is rather disgusting, but I was determined to pass this test and move on to real food. I give the rehab hospital credit, because the staff would reshape pureed green beans in a mold, so they actually looked like green beans. Same with the meat puree. They'd put it in a mold, and voila! It looked kind of like meat. The menu options were very slim.

"Would you like turkey, ham or beef puree?" they'd ask. I'd choose one, and it would come with mashed potatoes and a pureed vegetable. It helped if there was some sort of gravy. I would try to eat as much of the food on my plate as possible to also avoid supplemental tube feedings. After every meal, the PCTs would come in, see how much I'd eaten, and add up my calories. They said that if I didn't get enough calories, we'd have to use the tube.

I could not feed myself. I didn't yet have the arm strength to lift my hand to my mouth. We were working on it during OT, practicing with those beads and marbles in a bowl that I had to lift to my mouth on a spoon, but I hadn't yet regained the strength to accomplish this challenge. So I had to have someone there to feed me. My first meal came on January 24th, the morning after the swallow test. Jeff helped feed me the mush sent up from the kitchen. I was pretty ecstatic to eat "real" food, but I felt like a kid being fed by her parents. It was more than slightly awkward to open my mouth for food, and then try to tell my well-meaning husband to slow down. He was shoveling it in!

If Jeff or one of my friends was not there, then the PCT had to feed me. Unfortunately they had a lot of people to feed, so I would often wait for an hour to have my breakfast. You can imagine what mushy cold eggs taste like. I had been through worse things, so I bucked up and ate as much as I could. The threat of supplemental tube feedings in the back of my mind willed me to eat.

Once, Jeff came to my room with Doritos. It hit me; I had to have a Dorito. Doritos remind me of happy times. Every year I take a trip with my four best girlfriends, the BACH tribe. We always have Doritos. Laura Ball hates Doritos, so we like to eat them in front of her. Plus the rest of us are pretty darn good at finishing off a few bags. By the way, these are the amazing women who stayed many nights with me in the hospital, freezing their booties off because my room was kept as cold as possible. Not to mention it was the third coldest and snowiest Chicago winter on record. My friends who came to spend the night often slept in their winter coats. So I smiled when Jeff brought the bag of Doritos.

"I want one of those!" I told Jeff.

"Doritos do not qualify as pureed food," he said, so I had to use my great persuasion skills. He gave me the tiniest corner of a Dorito. I remember him putting it in my mouth. I let it sit on my tongue to soften a bit like babies do with those puff things. I had to really concentrate to swallow that Dorito, but it tasted like heaven!

"It's time for McDonald's French fries!" I told Jeff. Those fries are my Achilles heel. But that is all I wanted. My appetite was coming back, and they sounded so good. My awesome husband went out in the frigid temperatures, walked to McDonald's, and brought me back French fries and chicken nuggets. I probably had a total of five fries and a few nibbles of a chicken nugget, but those made me smile big! Life was slowly coming back.

January 31, 2014

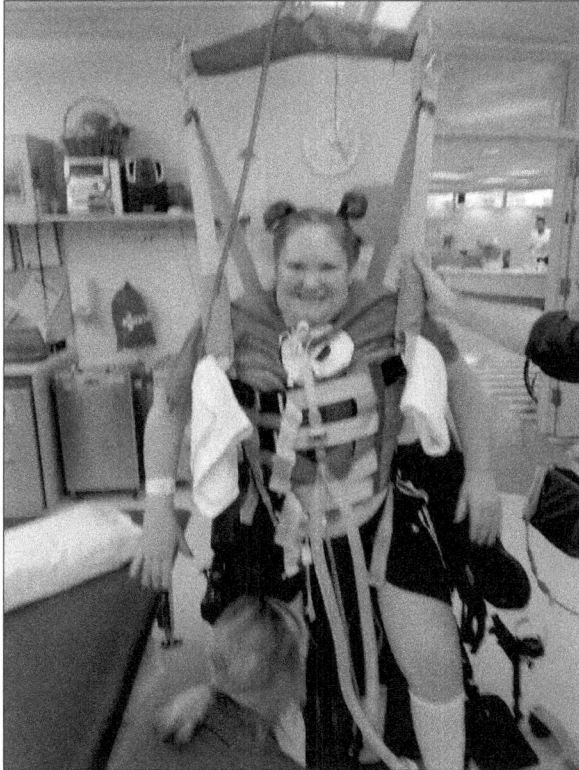

*Carrie standing for the first time in almost
two months.*

Fri, Jan 31, 2014 at 2:21 P.M., from Jeff's email:

Update for Friday, January 31st

Carrie's had a busy week of therapies. Scheduling has been up and down with therapists, so we have not yet had a chance to get fitted for a walking harness. She wore herself out pretty hard yesterday, so is very tired and sore today. She got some good news during speech however - her eating has been going so well that she has been upgraded to 'soft foods' so not everything has to be pureed mush.

She has worked very hard with her Occupational Therapists this week - grasping, holding, and moving her arms as much as she can. She's been very excited to do everything they ask. She's also very happy they rigged her up a long straw for drinking water during therapies.

She had some visitors this week and said it really helped to brighten up her days. So let me know if you'd like to come see her - hours are 8am-8pm every day but she usually has therapies until 3 or 4, so late afternoons are the best times.

Jeff

I was finally getting over the hump of feeling just plain crappy. Towards the end of January, I remember telling Jeff that I was starting to feel better and more like myself. I apologized for being grumpy while I'd felt so uncomfortable and hurt so much. Jeff told me I was a trooper and the grumpiness was completely understandable.

Once I cleared that hurdle and began to feel well, my therapy progress seemed to really speed up. About this time, I learned that Zoe, my favorite OT, who had been so encouraging, so caring, and just plain amazing, was taking a different job in the rehab hospital. I was moving to an OT named Anne Marie, who was seven months pregnant with twin boys! I was so bummed to be losing a therapist who had been so inspirational to me, but it turns out that Anne Marie was just as spectacular. She really pushed me to regain my ability to do those day-to-day tasks.

Since I was able to move my arms and fingers, it was essential that I use them as much as possible to regain strength and full range of motion. At first, my hands were so weak they couldn't grip anything. Now that I had the clearance to eat soft foods, I knew I had to get this holding a fork thing down. The therapists had all sorts of contraptions to help make daily tasks, like eating, independent. They gave me this rocker knife thing. To use it, I'd lightly grasp the handle and literally rock it back and forth to cut food on my plate. They also provided bent spoons and forks, which held food more easily, making it possible for me to get the utensils—and the food—into my mouth. I might be known for always spilling things on my shirt, and I lived up to that prestigious label when I was re-learning how to eat.

On January 31st, Jeff was at work, planning to come to the hospital late in the afternoon. My PT was anxious to get me up and walking in a harness contraption that helped bear my weight so I could work on walking, starting with movements that used my hips, legs, and ankles. Jeff was so excited to witness this with me, so all week we kept asking when it might happen. We were bummed to find out from Patrick that it would have to be next week because the walking lab was all booked. So Jeff stayed at work later that day.

Of course, after all the anticipation then disappointment, Patrick showed up in my room and said, "Let's go walk!"

Fortunately, by this point I was doing longer and longer periods of leak speech, so I could talk to Patrick during this adventure. Unfortunately, Jeff wasn't there to share it with me. I was scared and anxious to walk in the harness. What if it couldn't hold my weight? What if my legs just buckled?

The lab was on the tenth floor and had two machines to help patients walk. Patrick started putting two big straps around my thighs, using towels as pads to keep the straps from rubbing on my skin. Two more straps went up to my chest. These would be hooked to the machine. Getting the straps in place wasn't easy given that my legs were still so weak, but we did it! Then they pushed my 1,000-pound electric wheelchair up the ramp and start hooking up harnesses. Patrick explained that when I was ready, they would crank the harness pulleys to gradually lift me out of the wheelchair and get me in a standing position on a treadmill. Once I was in that position, he would start the treadmill on a very, very slow setting and he and Jill would help move my legs.

Did I mention I was terrified? So many thoughts flooded my mind. How did I end up in this position having to re-learn how to walk? What if my muscles never recovered? Then I started thinking, "Oh my gosh I am going to stand and take some steps. I wish Jeff was here!"

"Let's do this," Patrick said, and began cranking me up. I had brought my phone with me and I told Patrick we had to get this on video for Jeff.

I'm not going to sugarcoat it: the harness was not the most comfortable thing. Patrick had warned me about that and said if it's too much, we may be forced to stop.

"No way," I thought to myself. "I am pushing through any pain to get this walking party started." And then I was up! They took my blood pressure to make sure I was okay. With the nervousness and the sheer effort to get into position, I was already sweating. My blood pressure was good, so Patrick set the treadmill on slow and started it just as he and Jill each took hold of a leg, helping me pull it through a step motion and push off with the ball of my foot. It felt completely awkward and uncomfortable, but I was up and moving! I did not last long. I think I made it three minutes that first time. I remember sitting down and feeling so tired, but I had to get up and do it again. This was going to be hard work, but it was the best way to get back to walking as quickly as I could.

The next try, we got on video. I love that I had these videos showing the first time I "walked" as I recovered from GBS. I gave thumbs up on the video. I was proud of myself! I was super bummed that Jeff missed it, but I couldn't wait to show him the video when he arrived a few hours later.

He started to tear up as he watched. It was almost like seeing your child walk for the first time. Jeff was so relieved to see me up. He told me months later that when we were at Northwestern Memorial Hospital, the neurologist had pulled him aside and said, "I need to paint you the potential worst, so you are prepared. There is a good chance your wife may never walk again. It is too early to tell, but she has many of the telltale signs that a full recovery may not happen." Apparently being on a vent more than two weeks is rare. Additionally, paralysis going all the way up to the eyes is often a sign that a patient's case is so severe that full recovery is difficult, and probably unlikely. Jeff cried that day I walked because he knew I was beating those odds.

The other huge turning point that week was being allowed to have water whenever I wanted. I still could not lift a glass of water by myself, so my occupational therapist, Anne Marie, rigged up a straw mechanism with Doreen. It was like a super-duper long straw that kids would love. They put it in my water and it was hooked up so that I could move my head to the side and reach it to get a drink. The freedom to drink water! You have no idea how refreshing this achievement was. I no longer had to beg my friends or Jeff to dip the sponge into the ice-cold water and let me suck on it to get water into my mouth. I started drinking lots of water (which also brought about a lot of peeing).

Until you are in that kind of situation, you don't really want to think about how going to the bathroom works. I've already described the bed pan ordeal. When I had to pee, I would have to go back to my room, get them to take me out of my wheelchair, put me back in bed and then they would have to roll me over to put a bed pan under me.

Why not roll me into the bathroom, you're wondering? Well, I wasn't able to scoot over on a transfer board to the toilet yet. I didn't have enough arm strength to get there. There was no good way for me to use a toilet in my condition. The positive thing was that I could feel when I needed to pee. I could tell the nurses when I needed their help. I got pretty darn good at holding my pee as I often had to wait for a PCT and nurse to have time to come in to help me. Unfortunately, my ability to tell when I had to go number two had not fully recovered yet.

"How come you are still using a bed pan?" One of my favorite nurses and PCT asked one night. "You can use the women's urinal."

I had not heard of such a thing. I was fascinated and completely interested. (Let's face it – guys have it much easier when it comes to peeing while lying in a bed. Someone brings in a urinal bottle and they get the job done. Women are not built that conveniently.) The women's urinal looked like a tall skinny pitcher. They would place it right next to my privates and I would try to get my pee in the opening. Some nurses and PCTs were pros at the exact angle and position to hold it... others not so much. When I could talk, I would encourage them to put pads underneath me—the kind they use to clean up number twos or put under you in bed to prevent messes. Sorry! I know this may be a bit graphic, but I think it's important to understand how hard some of this is so if you or a family member find yourself in the situation, you'll understand it is all completely normal. There is nothing fun nor private about it, but you come to realize you have no choice.

Since peeing was such an ordeal, I often held out as long as I could before I gave in to the need. I know, I know, that's not good for you and can result in urinary tract infections. Fortunately, I never had to deal with one of those at RIC. The women's urinal was amazing in that it let us skip the steps of rolling me onto one side, rolling me back onto the bedpan, then rolling me off of the bedpan without spilling it. With the urinal, I would lie on my back and they would move my head up a bit to have gravity assist in the process. The only problem with the urinal was I peed a lot. No, seriously: I filled that thing up at least five times. I had to try to stop mid-stream so they could empty it and come back. Talk about Kegel exercises. The nurses and PCTs were always stunned at how much I peed. It was because I was so excited to finally be able to drink water.

Going number two wasn't nearly as fun. They had this thing called the bowel program. Individuals who have spinal cord injuries have difficulty releasing their bowels. I was on the spinal cord injury floor at RIC, where almost everyone was on the bowel program. I am not sure how I avoided it the month of January, but one day one of my nurses told me he was going to recommend a bowel program to my doctor. It had been a rough day of accidents—imagine your worst nightmare when you turn older and have to wear adult diapers. That was me! Controlling my bowels was iffy at best. Usually by the time I realized I had to go, there was no hope of actually getting out of my wheelchair, moved to my bed, and rolled onto a bedpan in time. I usually had a bowel movement every two or three days. If I hadn't gone after three days, they'd threaten stool softeners and other fun stuff.

Brooke was there the night they told me I was joining the bowel program. Ironically, I was pissed. It was a dumb idea and I didn't want to do it. Who really wants a suppository, which will make you poop in bed (while lying on pads to catch the poo)? Super fun! Brooke was on my side and told me I had every right to resist. I was in charge of my care. I remember debating it and weighing the pros and cons. The pros: I would get my body back on a normal schedule I could control. It also meant I wouldn't get stopped up. The cons: Well, I think I pretty much already laid those out for you. But my stomach hurt because I hadn't pooped in a few days, and so I said, "What they heck – I will try it once." It helped that one of my favorite nurses, Julia, was helping me that night. I asked her a ton of questions then asked her opinion. She was supportive of my decision to give it a "go." It was not a pleasant process whatsoever, but I got into a routine and made the best out of the situation. I decided that I would pick a TV show I hadn't yet seen, and watch that show on my iPad while I was doing my bowel program. That is when I started watching *House of Cards*. Politicians and shit… the irony is not lost on me. (Note to Mom: of course, not *all* politicians should get a bad rap.)

January 31, 2014 Addendum

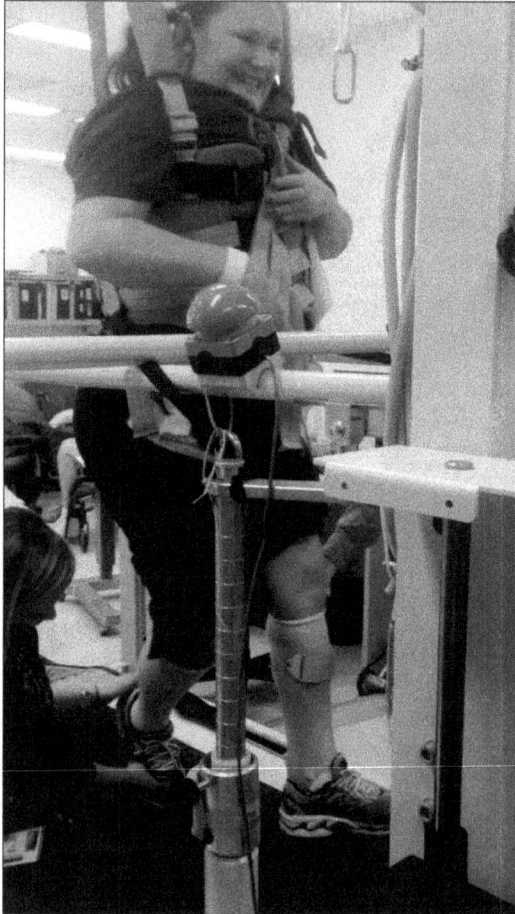

Carrie walking on the treadmill for the first time!

Fri, Jan 31, 2014 at 5:44 p.m., from Jeff's email:

Exciting Addendum for Friday night

Carrie had late PT today and her therapists decided today was the day. They got her up into the harness and she stood up assisted for twenty-five minutes! She even took several assisted steps. She did amazing. The therapists were worried that she'd have a lot of leg pain since she's been so sensitive! She did amazingly well and is very excited to progress. I've attached a few pics to show you all. She's doing so well—did even more OT by driving her chair around the floor. Somehow the speed keeps getting set to 'rabbit' and she just takes off. Lots of fun when I'm the guy who pushes the vent behind!

Jeff

You've read Jeff's story of me walking for the first time. It was a glorious day and I think that was the first night I saw Jeff smile really big! I was also progressing in driving my chair. (Jeff's note also mentioned this achievement. As usual, he never missed a chance to sing my praises.) At this point, the feeling was coming back in my hands so I could use the joystick to steer the wheelchair! While my hands were attempting to steer my wheelchair (which was not always a fluid motion), I would sometimes accidentally change the speed. I still had to have someone follow me up and down the hallway with my vent. I was getting tired of dragging that thing around. I was pushing each day to go off the vent for longer and longer periods, but if I left the room, it still had to go with me. I also still had to be suctioned, so I had to take all of that fun gear with me as well. It was getting old.

I pushed my respiratory therapists, asking them when we could go without the ventilator. They cautioned me not to rush it, but promised we would try soon. During the day they worried about me being off the vent when I napped. When we sleep, our muscles relax, which can cause oxygen levels to drop. I was still sleeping quite a lot at this stage. I would come back from an especially busy day of therapy, crash, and take a nap before dinner. They started weaning me off the vent a bit every day but would put me back on the vent if I wanted to nap. We were working to build up my stamina.

One day I accidentally fell asleep, and I did fine that first time sleeping off the vent! I was scared to tell anyone I had fallen asleep for fear they were going to make me go back on the vent immediately. If my oxygen had dropped, my monitor would have gone off, and it didn't. Another milestone in the book! That vent was on my short list of things to overcome!

February 5, 2014

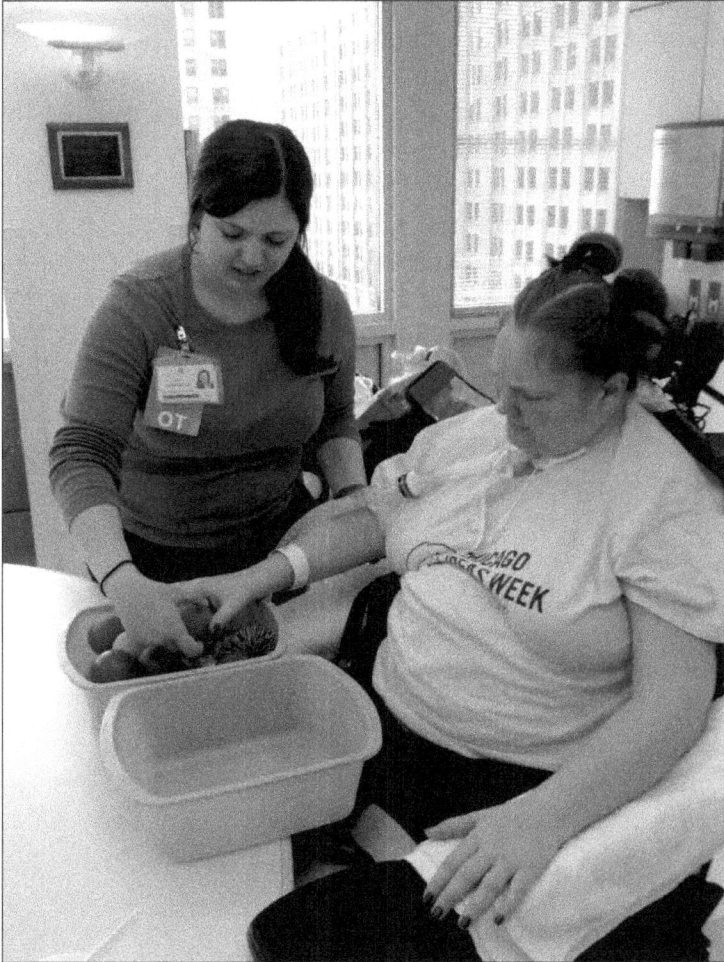

Carrie in occupational therapy trying to grip balls.

Feb 5, 2014 at 5:29 p.m., from **Jeff's email**:

Update for Wednesday, February 5ᵗʰ

This week thus far has been a bit of a struggle. Carrie had a bad headache on Monday, and yesterday had a chest x-ray because the respiratory folks and her doctor were concerned about her losing her voice. The x-ray came back normal, lungs and chest are all clear. The concern is that there's something blocking her trachea above the tube but below her vocal cords, preventing her speech and making leak speech not leaky. The end result is no leak speech until she sees the ENT doc, most likely on a day trip back over to Northwestern, and we probably won't see him until Tuesday. The most likely possible causes are an inflammation of the cords themselves, or some kind of scar tissue growth resulting from the tracheostomy surgery.

So she's understandably bummed about not speaking for five or six days, but she's still making great strides on her OT and PT, and speech cleared her for thin liquids, which means she can drink whatever she wants, whenever she wants. The only thing remaining for food is hard solids—pills, tortilla chips, hard crackers, raw veggies, etc. That's on the slate for next week.

She did several OT tests with her arm strength and dexterity today—on a scale of one to fifty-seven, she scored a forty-three right and a thirty-three left—hugely improved from three weeks ago when she couldn't even lift her right hand.

She's looking forward to those of you planning to visit, but come with stories because she won't be talking for a few days!

Jeff

This voice issue was a setback. I was not a happy camper to have gotten back the gift of my voice, my personality, my ability to communicate then bam! It was gone. My trachea was definitely one of the reasons my patience grew immensely while I was sick. It was out of my control—my body had ideas other than the recovery path I had in my head. I was forced to adapt. I had to adjust my expectations and remind myself, "I survived not talking before, I can do it again." It was incredibly frustrating as well that the ENT doctor did not come daily, but weekly, and only if we were lucky. If he had an emergency at the hospital, he didn't come to RIC. As someone desperately waiting to see the doctor, I really did not appreciate being stood up.

My OT, Anne Marie, introduced me to tests for my hand strength. I remember the first time she had me do it. I am maybe one of the most competitive people you will meet. To be given the Action Research Arm Test (ARAT) test and barely score a thirty-three (yes, I rounded up), of the test goal of fifty-seven (I know: random scale for a test, right?) pained me! The first part of the test consisted of picking up blocks and marbles and placing them in a dish. Next, she pulled out little silver balls that looked like BB gun ammo. There was no way in hell I could pick up a tiny silver ball. Then I had to pour water from one cup into another cup. My hand was shaking badly but I did it! I was elated just to hold the glass. This meant I might be able to hold my own cup of water! I convinced Anne Marie we had to work on that later that day.

Anne Marie got me. She knew I was competitive and internally driven. She created a chart for my room with my initial scores and a big star by fifty-seven—the highest score you can achieve. Everyone who came into my room would ask about the graphs and what I was working on. It was a huge motivator and as my scores advanced, I was so proud. When Jeff arrived, I'd tell him right away to look at the graphs. I knew he'd share my joy when he saw my progress. It was the little things like increasing my scores on that test that kept me going!

February 9, 2014

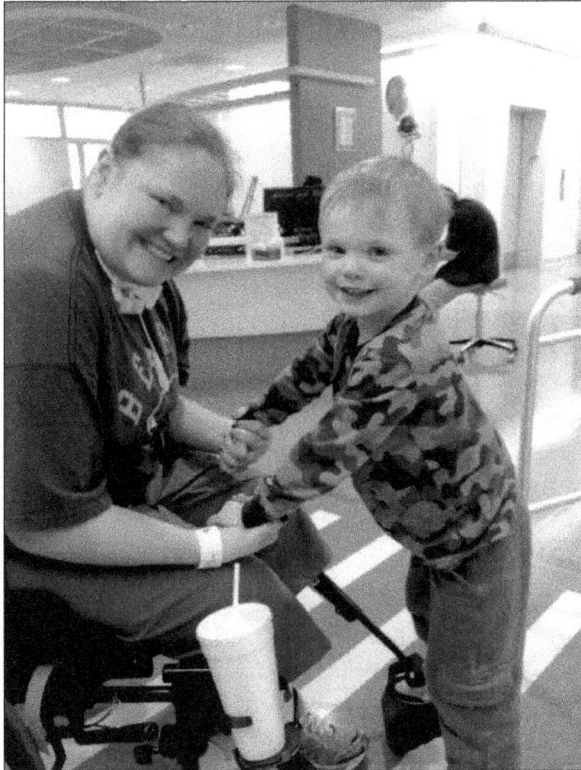

Carrie in her wheelchair holding Will's hand,
water cup by her side!

Sun, Feb 9, 2014 at 7:15 p.m., from **Jeff's email**:

Update for Sunday, February 9th

We're still waiting confirmation from Northwestern for Carrie's ENT appointment. Hopefully we're still on for Tuesday and get this figured out.

Carrie is making awesome progress on all other fronts. The last several days she has been staying completely off her vent for longer and longer periods of time. Four hours on Thursday, six on Friday and Saturday, and thus far today she's gone ten hours nonstop. So we are very hopeful that we'll be coming off of the vent for good soon!

She's also made great strides with her arms. Will came to visit today and she was able to give him a hug. She had the biggest smile I've seen in a while. Her PT today also got her up in the walking harness. Making those legs go is a lot of work but she did amazing—no problems breathing, and her pulse rate stayed steady as well.

Hope to have more good news to report after Tuesday. Thanks to all who came and visited over the weekend, she really appreciated beating all of you at Wii table tennis!

Sun, Feb 9, 2014 at 7:16 p.m., from **Jeff's email**:
PS - Thank you to all who have sent flowers and other gifts. I am so far behind on thank you notes. We appreciate all of your generosity and support!

The rehab hospital had a day room with a large TV and a Nintendo Wii. Sometimes for OT I got to Wii bowl. Using the Wii remote let me work on my grip and, when I was able, I would stand and work on my balance. When you are just getting your hand strength back, holding a remote is hard. I wore the wrist straps to make sure I didn't fling the remote into the TV.

One Friday, I'd had a busy afternoon of PT and OT. I had hoped for a lower-key day. I was tired. As I got ready to get in my wheelchair to go to PT, a familiar face appeared at my door. It was Hrishi! If you knew Hrishi, you would be smiling right now. Hrishi, who is from India, and I met in college at Purdue. We really became friends when I interviewed and then brought him out to my client site when we both worked in consulting after college. Hrishi has a deep Hindi accent so I usually have to pause and really listen to what he is saying. No matter what he is saying, though, he exudes passion and excitement! As they started to put me in my sling and lift me to my wheelchair, Hrishi was yelling "Carrie Campbell (my maiden name)! What are they doing?" For someone who had not seen me be moved into my wheelchair it was quite the spectacle! Once I was in my chair, I showed off my driving skills. The entire ten minutes was quite funny. I still couldn't talk, so communicating with Hrishi was very difficult. I just smiled a lot!

We headed into PT and I introduced Hrishi to Patrick and Jill. Hrishi makes friends instantly. People were slapping him on the back and asking him for stories about me. Next thing you know, Hrishi's sidekick, Osamu, comes strolling in. Osamu, aka Sam, worked in consulting with us. I had spent many workdays and then nights out with these two jokesters. When you put Hrishi and Sam together, laughter is sure to erupt. My PT had me up in the harness walking, showing off for Hrishi and Sam. Then I was sitting on the edge of the padded table and we were playing balloon volleyball. Hrishi and Sam were telling everyone jokes and had all the patients and therapists laughing.

Next up was OT. It was our lucky day as my OT suggested we do a little Nintendo Wii. So I took Sam on in Wii bowling! Unfortunately, he was a rock star in the bowling arena and kicked my bootie. (I need to challenge Sam to a rematch now that I have all of my strength back!) It was a super afternoon with my friends and reminded me of the life I had ahead of me to enjoy.

Then on Sunday Will came to visit. That made my week! Will's bright smiling face always lifted my spirits. He lit up the room and everyone loved to see him. The day I finally got to hug him—after two months of just having to watch him, mouth "I love you," and wave to him—I could not wait to put my arms around him and cuddle. Hugging their children isn't only lovely, it's a necessity for moms. Cuddling is essential for physical and emotional well-being. Luckily Will got lots of hugs and cuddles from dad and his grandparents while Mom was in the hospital. Will was always so proud of me when I would have a new trick to show him. One week it was winking at him, another it was moving my shoulders, then it was moving my head, next lifting my arm off the bed—and now hugging him!

He would usually come and sit on my bed and watch his iPad. Just having him near made me smile. Then he would want me to get in my wheelchair so he could watch me drive around. For that, I got to be off the ventilator a few hours, so I didn't have all the tubes to drag with me. Without all that paraphernalia, I think Will was starting to see his old mom come back to him.

Feb 10, 2014 4:40 p.m., from Jeff's email:

Quick note while I have a free moment

Carrie's appointment with the ENT at Northwestern is 'on the schedule' for Wednesday. We do not yet know what time, or where the procedure will be performed (OR or procedure room), but in theory we're the first appointment of the day and should be back at RIC in the afternoon. So keep us in your thoughts and prayers Wednesday morning!

February 12, 2014

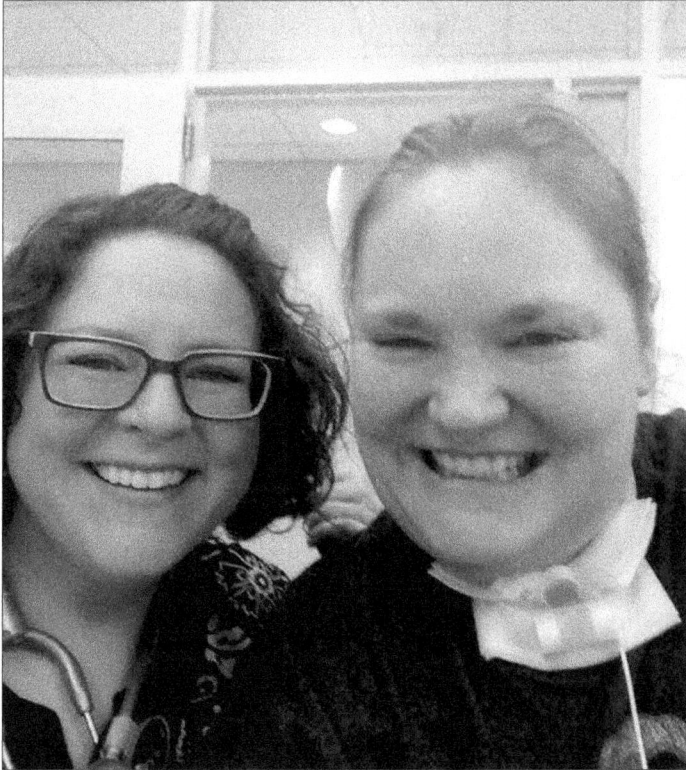

Carrie and nurse Julia.

Wed, Feb 12, 2014 at 7:24 p.m., from **Jeff's email**:

Update for Wednesday February 12th

Carrie's surgery was a success today. We arrived at Northwestern around 7:30 a.m. and procedure started around 9:20. She was in recovery for about two hours and we made it back to RIC by 2:00 p.m. The ENT told me it was what he expected, granulation around the trach tube. He was able to clean it up by cryo-laser, which I think is pretty sweet. We hope Carrie will get her voice back tomorrow, but it may take another day. He also mentioned that there is a possibility this can reoccur while she has a tube in, so recommended we get off the vent ASAP. Carrie says she's ready to go as soon as they'll let her. Today is the fifth full day of being off the vent all day. They knocked her out completely for the procedure and she breathed just fine, so next steps are to try a night without vent and see how we do then either go to a smaller tube or a different type. Last step is obviously to pull the tubes and sew them up.

Will update more this weekend.

Jeff

I remember going over to Northwestern for surgery in early February. They came really early in the morning to pick me up. I still didn't have feeling in my legs, so they had to transport me by ambulance. You don't realize how difficult situations like prepping for surgery are when you do not have full mobility. I had to give a urine sample to make sure I wasn't pregnant. Seriously? Did we mention I have been at the rehab hospital for more than a month? I was not alone even to pee most days so I am not sure where they thought we would fit in a little naked tango. I guess Jeff looks like a sex-driven husband. Just kidding! The nurses did tell us that we would be surprised how often they catch people doing it in hospitals! Crazy.

This was the first time throughout the entire ordeal that I understood ahead of time what to expect, so it was a bit scary. They were going to put me under, so the anesthesiologist came in and asked a ton of questions. I was pretty tired of retelling my story and since I still could not talk… Jeff got to do all the talking! The doctor's entourage (that is how I referred to the interns and residents) talked me through the procedure. Then the doctor came by to make sure I did not have any questions. I, of course, did have a few questions which I relayed via Jeff.

And it was time to go to surgery. They put a hospital cap on my head, gave me something to take the edge off, and wheeled me away. The surgical room was cold. Nurses and residents were talking and setting stuff up. It was a bit overwhelming. They moved me to the operating table and asked if I was ready to go to sleep. But wait—

"Where is the doctor?" someone asked.

There was a quick scramble to track him down to make sure they didn't put me to sleep before he was ready. The doctor walked in the door and they could begin.

Next thing I knew, I woke up in recovery. I had some pain. I remember waking for a minute and then falling back asleep. My head hurt. The nurse asked if I wanted pain medicine. "YES!" I mouthed. A few hours later, they let Jeff see me then we headed back to RIC. We were re-loaded into the ambulance to travel literally two-tenths of a mile. I slept on and off for the afternoon. We were all hopeful my voice would come back by the next day!

February 17, 2014

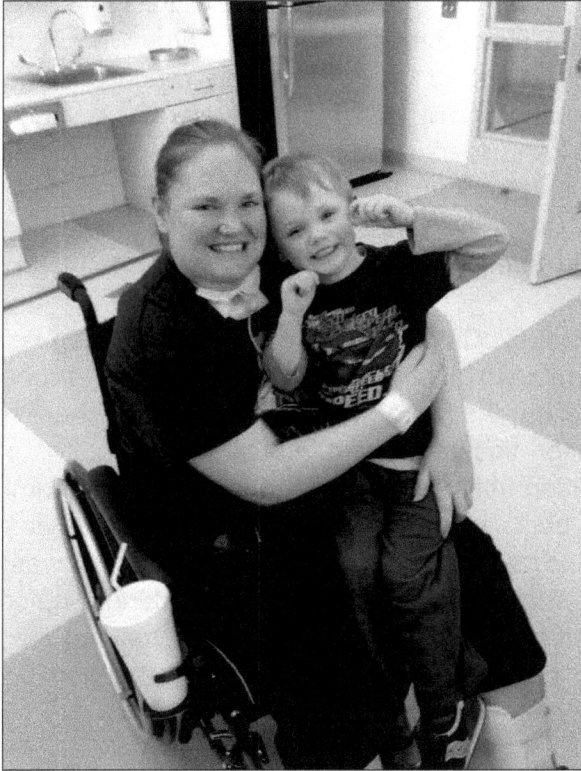

Carrie with Will on her lap.

Mon, Feb 17, 2014 at 5:48 p.m., from **Jeff's email**:

Update for Monday February 17th

Carrie had a pretty good weekend. Her physical rehab continues to progress very well. Today she was able to get up on a treadmill with her physical therapist and take several harness-assisted steps. Andy and Kathy were here for the long weekend and I know she very much enjoyed seeing and spending time with them. Will and I came down on Saturday and spent a couple of hours playing games, eating snacks and hanging out in Mom's chair. We had a pretty good Valentine's dinner as well with some sushi and sparkling cider.

Unfortunately, Carrie's voice continues to be an issue. She is still unable to talk around the trach so there is concern that the swelling has not gone down and/or there is more granulation tissue growing in. The ENT doctor is also now on vacation until next Monday, so she's pretty bummed. To further bum everyone out, the outing she was looking forward to the Museum of Science and Industry was also put on hold due to the concerns about speaking. She continues to breathe perfectly well off the ventilator, but the doctors want to be absolutely safe with the breathing so they're being very cautious.

She is able to text now on her phone and loves to hear from you so if you want to "chat" with her that's about the best way. I'll update later this week as we know more.

My voice didn't come back after the first surgery. Then the ENT doctor went on vacation. When Jeff broke that news to me, I lost it. I was hanging out in the day room and I just started sobbing. I think it shocked quite a few of the patients and therapists who happened to be there. They had rarely seen me cry. They knew me as a positive person who had a good outlook throughout my situation. But on this day, I just could not muster the energy to overcome this setback. I needed a pity party. That went on for about fifteen minutes—me crying, Jeff reassuring me, rubbing my back, and telling me that our surviving the past two months meant that we would get through this, too. He was right. I bucked up, pulled myself together, and went on to my scheduled physical therapy.

I was making more and more progress with physical therapy. I was able to handle being on my legs in the harness longer and longer. Patrick was pushing me, and I was meeting all of the goals he set in front of me.

So right before Valentine's Day the RIC staff informed me that I was moving to a new room. The good news: it was right next door. The bad news: I would have a roommate. At RIC there were twenty-eight rooms on a floor and only four were individual rooms. They have now built a new state-of-the-art hospital with more individual rooms, which is how most hospitals are today. Since I was off the ventilator and making progress on my recovery, I was no longer in need of an individual room. They reserved those rooms for high-risk ventilator patients and those requiring more attention. Fortunately, my roommate was a likeable young woman about my age. (Notice I threw "young" in there?) Betty (not her real name) was in a wheelchair permanently. I don't remember what caused her injury, but she had a son who was about eight or nine, and a boyfriend who came to visit her only every few weeks since they didn't live in Illinois. She was at RIC for a program called "second chance." Patients who had previously been at RIC could come back and get physical and occupational therapy to help expand their abilities. Betty was a sweetheart who was very easy to live with.

Valentine's weekend was fun because my mom and brother visited. (My dad was on a scuba-diving trip.) My brother always provided good humor and commentary.

"If you wanted to lose weight, you could have just gone on a diet" or "If you needed a break from work, there are other ways!" I expected nothing less from Andy, who is a master of sarcasm.

It was really good to see my mom. It had been almost a month since her last visit. She was so excited to see the progress I had made from the last time she had seen me in the ICU. I had come so far, being able to move and raise my arms, eating, breathing on my own most of the day—she found it phenomenal that I could do all of these "simple" tasks." At the time, I remember still feeling frustrated, longing for my life before I was sick. I wanted to be at my house, sleeping in my bed, playing with Will, and having a normal routine to my life. That end still seemed pretty far away, but when people came to visit me who had seen me at my worst in the ICU, and they could see my progress, they helped me see it too. This was HUGE! It was essential to celebrate all of those small wins along the way. It helped keep it all in perspective. It could be worse, I knew.

On Valentine's Day, we ordered sushi, and I ate a few pieces. Food still didn't taste normal and I just wasn't hungry. We also ordered a few Chinese dishes. As Andy was passing a dish to me, I dropped it all over the floor. My dexterity wasn't back to normal yet. I was making huge improvement, but I was not yet fully there! I felt bad and I could tell my brother was bummed, but he handled it well. He said not one word, just quietly cleaned it up. We were all so happy to be hanging out together—a little dropped food could not get us down.

I think Jeff was a little disappointed that we didn't get to be together, just the two of us, on Valentine's Day. We have a tradition that on Valentine's Day we stay home and cook something unique. One year it was shabu-shabu, another year fondue, another crab legs. This Valentine's Day I was so thankful for Jeff and the fact I had him in my life. When you get married, you never know one hundred percent if it will work. There are no guarantees in life or in relationships. I definitely got lucky meeting and marrying Jeff!

We got a chuckle out of my mother's ability to do my hair that weekend. When I was growing up, my mom was not the type to do my hair. We relied on my friend's mom who was a beautician to braid my hair for softball games and to fix my hair for dances. So, when my mom visited that weekend, I asked her if she would put my hair up in pigtails like the nurses did for me. That was the best hair do to sleep in. It got my hair up so it was not so hot with it on my neck. No surprise, my mom struggled to get my hair in pigtails. She must have tried three or four times before she called it good enough. Later that morning Anne Marie, my OT, walked into the day room.

"Who fixed your hair today?" she asked. "It looks awful!"

Anne Marie proceeded to take it out and re-do it. My mom handled that with grace. We giggled about it later.

The day before Valentine's Day, I reached a major milestone: I went all night without the ventilator. Another

HUGE achievement! Jeff and I had spent hours having conversations with the respiratory teams at Northwestern Memorial Hospital and RIC about weaning me off the ventilator. Everyone had a different opinion, and no one wanted to make promises. If you remember, they'd originally tried to wean me off of the vent before we left the NMH ICU. It was unsuccessful, and they thought it would be better to get me to the rehab hospital to get therapy started and try to wean me off later. When we arrived at RIC, they explained they do not wean people off ventilators. Jeff and I were thoroughly confused because no one seemed to be able to tell us how the process would really work. Ultimately, with the help of a few of the respiratory therapists at RIC, Jeff and I got it done. We were determined.

It was difficult and scary at first, when they suctioned but wouldn't give me breaths in between. It was conditioning (like working out) for my lungs and body, and most importantly, my mind. It freaked me out at first, but over time, I became more and more comfortable and that is how I eventually got to February 13th when I was off the vent a full 24 hours! I was done. They kept that ventilator in my room for a few days, just in case. I told all of my therapists my idea on what to do with that vent. Do you remember the scene from the movie *Office Space* when they take the printer out to the field and take a few baseball bats to it? That was what I thought should be done to the vent. Forget the fact that the vent was rented so, technically, I didn't own it. Both Patrick and Anne Marie thought my suggestion was hilarious.

So on Valentine's Day, my mom, brother Jeff, and I celebrated the end of the vent! I am pretty sure Jeff cried. The doctors at NMH had told Jeff I may never come off the vent.

Another doctor from RIC told me a few days later that he did not think I would get off the vent. He had told my therapists that, too. I loved proving them all wrong and beating the odds!

Being off was such a relief. I no longer had to bring it along when I took off in my wheelchair. A nurse just had to get me out of bed, then I was in charge. I could take off wherever I wanted! I felt so free—like a kid going off to college! Freedom!

I was sad to see my mom and brother leave that weekend. I wasn't able to talk, but they got a lot better at reading my lips that weekend! Jeff was the very best lip reader, but most people picked it up if they spent a few days with me. There were key things (water, pain meds, massages, etc.) that I always asked for, so that made it easier.

My mom was hoping to see me next when I was home! She was a Nebraska state senator at the time, and was planning to come back when the legislative session was over and stay with us for an extended period. I always cried when my mom left. There is something about having your mom around when you don't feel good that is just so reassuring.

February 24, 2014

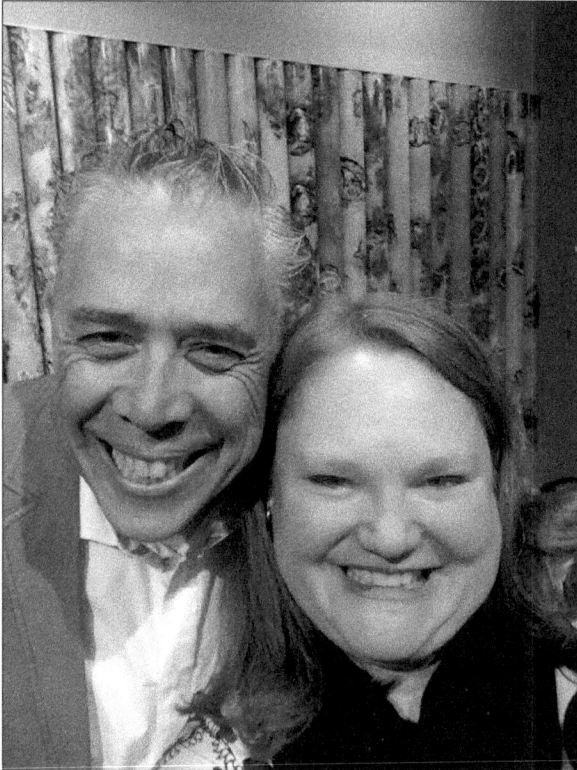

*Carrie and Dan Spencer a few years after GBS
celebrating Kathy's (Carrie's mom's) retirement.*

Mon, Feb 24, 2014 at 8:18 p.m., from **Jeff's email**:

Update for Monday, February 24th

Carrie had another good weekend. We enjoyed seeing her pseudo-brother, Dan Spencer. He flew in and spent the weekend in Chicago hanging out with Carrie.

Today she had a pretty awesome breakthrough—she got up out of her chair on the parallel bars with no harness, only a therapist helping her up and steadying her hips! Making huge strides forward on the therapy fronts. She also retested the ARAT score and put that sucker to bed— maximum scores on both arms and hands. Every time I go home for a night and come back, it seems like she's gotten stronger in some way!

To go with our new room, we have a new roommate who's unfortunately not quite as cool as her old roomie. We bought Carrie some noise-canceling headphones and that's helped a bit. Not really a big deal since most of the time she's up in her chair during the day when not in therapy. I think she's tired of hanging out in bed!

Tomorrow will also be a big day. We are scheduled to see an ENT doc here at RIC who can hopefully tell us more about what's going on with the speech and trach tube in general. We're hoping for at least a plan of attack if not a solution. I'll try to send an update again soon!

Jeff

It was great to see Dan's face! Dan lived with my family while he went to dental school when I was in my later years of elementary school and early days of junior high. In exchange for room and board in our home, Dan drove me to school, and to sports practices, and made sure Andy and I were fed on the nights my parents had to be gone. Dan witnessed some of the important experiences of my childhood, such as the day I brought my new flute home and cried when I couldn't figure out how to play it. Dan figured out how to teach a sobbing fifth-grade girl how to pucker her lips just the right way to play her new musical instrument. He was a big brother to me. He flew in from Colorado, taking time away from Sarah and their two children, to spend the weekend with me at RIC.

Dan was a great PT partner; he didn't give me any slack. He was there when I was working with Anne Marie on getting dressed. I had this grabber thing that I would use to act as my arm because I did not have the ability to move my body and arms in a coordinated fashion so I could pull up my pants or tie my shoes.

"Are you sure you cannot just lean over and do that?" Dan asked.

I laughed, but at one point he was right. I was trying to do something with the grabber thingy when I could have pushed myself to lean to the side a bit and do it naturally. It was so frustrating that a few short months ago I was a normal person, getting myself dressed in the morning without thinking twice. Now I was sweating profusely just trying to get my darn yoga pants pulled above my knees.

Will came to visit that Saturday and he was excited to hang out with Dan. Those dentists are pretty good at making glove balloons and other creations with doctors' gloves. Will enjoyed playing a little balloon volleyball with Dan in the day room. We played other games and hung out. As with so many passages on this journey, there was a drawback: I was still unable to talk. For Dan—a newcomer to my hospital room—reading lips was hard. I was able to use my fingers to type on my phone, so I was able to spell out a few things for him.

Roommates are tough to deal with when you are used to your own room and space, especially when you do not feel well. A change in roommates is an adjustment. Adjusting to my new roommate, Ellen (not her real name), was a challenge. The day Ellen moved in, I was at therapy and Jeff was in my room, working. He knew immediately that there was going to be trouble. Ellen and her family came flying in with her stuff, arguing, yelling, and cursing, and Ellen shouting for pain meds. The days of my nice, friendly roommate were over. Ellen was a woman I would guess to be in her mid-fifties. Her family lived about thirty minutes west of downtown Chicago but only visited her once a week. Based on comments she made to us, we believe she may have been a recovering drug addict. She was very loud and liked to talk a lot...to anyone who would listen. She was always asking for her pain medication hours before it was due. If the nurses were not able to come right away, she would moan...very loudly, then start yelling.

Ellen talked to me even though I was unable to talk back to her. I would have my TV on, and Ellen would be talking away. Then one day, she yelled "Clap if you hear me!" I was not sure I heard her correctly, then she yelled it again. "Clap if you hear me!" So I clapped, hoping she would be appeased and leave me alone. Nope—bad move on my part because now she would ask me quite regularly to "Clap if you are there and okay." One time I did not clap back, and Ellen started to freak out, called the nurses, yelling for them to check on me. I have to give her credit for her big heart and for watching out for me. Her tactics were just a bit much.

Ellen also fell asleep with her TV on full blast. I mean it was LOUD, just like her. I would often ask the nurses or PCTs to turn her TV off when I knew she was asleep so it wouldn't keep me up at night. I went from sleeping twelve hours a night in my own room, to barely getting five to six hours of sleep due to Ellen. That was not healthy for me, so I got on the internet and ordered myself some noise-cancelling headphones. I got a lot of strange looks from the night nurses, PCTs, and respiratory therapists! They would come in my room and start talking to me. I would not be able to hear them, so they would have to tap me on my shoulder to wake me up. Then they would point at my headphones, point to Ellen's bed, and chuckle. I think of Ellen every time I use those headphones today.

Despite the hassle of adjusting to a new roommate, my journey was positive in other ways. I was much more mobile now that I didn't have to travel everywhere with my ventilator, suction machine, and kits. I felt like a free woman! If Ellen started talking, I would ring for the nurses to get me out of bed. I would leave the room as early as I could after eating breakfast and I would not come back until the nurses would ask me to get into bed around 8:00 or 9:00 p.m. I spent a lot of time in the day room, conversing with other patients. Even though I could not talk much I could hang out. I would watch TV, listen to music, read on my iPad, or just snooze. I had a recline feature on my wheelchair that allowed me to lay almost flat. It was great for taking pressure off my tailbone and catching a quick nap! I think this is how I formed stronger relationships with the PCTs and nurses since they would come to the day room to get water or just to take a break.

My friend Megan also came the weekend that Dan was visiting. Megan had just had a baby and it was so great to see her and hear how her new daughter was doing. It was always interesting to have friends come visit who I had not seen while I was sick. You could see their shock at seeing their friend in a wheelchair, unable to talk, and not quite the person they knew and loved. As the visit went on, I could sense my friends start to be more comfortable as they realized the person they knew was inside of this body that had failed her. And I think most of them believed I was going to get better. All of those positive vibes were an important part of my recovery. It was a web of support that enveloped me.

Before Dan left to go home that weekend, he got to witness a first for me: I stood! I had walked on the treadmill while in a harness, but I had not yet stood and supported myself with my own strength. Therapists would roll my wheelchair in between parallel bars in the gym. Then they would put a gait belt around my hips. This thick belt gave them some leverage on my body, to keep me from falling.

"I think we can get you up to stand," the PT I was working with that day said.

"Okay! Let's try it!" I responded.

I had watched other patients stand up at the parallel bars, now it was my turn. In less than two months I had gone from being completely paralyzed and unable to move anything to getting ready to stand! I had not even been able to hold my own head up when they had first helped me out of my wheelchair. Now I could sit on a mat in the gym and had the core muscles to hold myself upright. I had taken steps on the treadmill and today I was going to try to stand up. I was so proud of myself.

My PT told me she was going to count to three and then I would stand up. She said to push through my arms with the parallel bars.

"One... two... three."

I pushed with all the might in my legs and with my arms. That first time the PT really helped pull me out of my chair, but I was standing. She even asked me to shift my weight from foot to foot and I could do that with a lot of effort and concentration. Since I still could not feel my legs or my feet, it was hard to tell if what my brain was telling them to do was actually working!

Dan was pumped and shot a video of the moment. After about twenty seconds, I told the PT I needed to sit down, and she slowly helped lower me into my chair. At that moment the room erupted in congratulations and clapping. I was completely unaware of it, but everyone had stopped their therapies to watch and cheer me on! I had a lot of fans in the other patients and therapists. I smiled from ear to ear and got a little choked up. I had just achieved this monumental step AND I had so much support getting to this point. You had to celebrate milestones like this because each day was so hard.

February 25, 2014

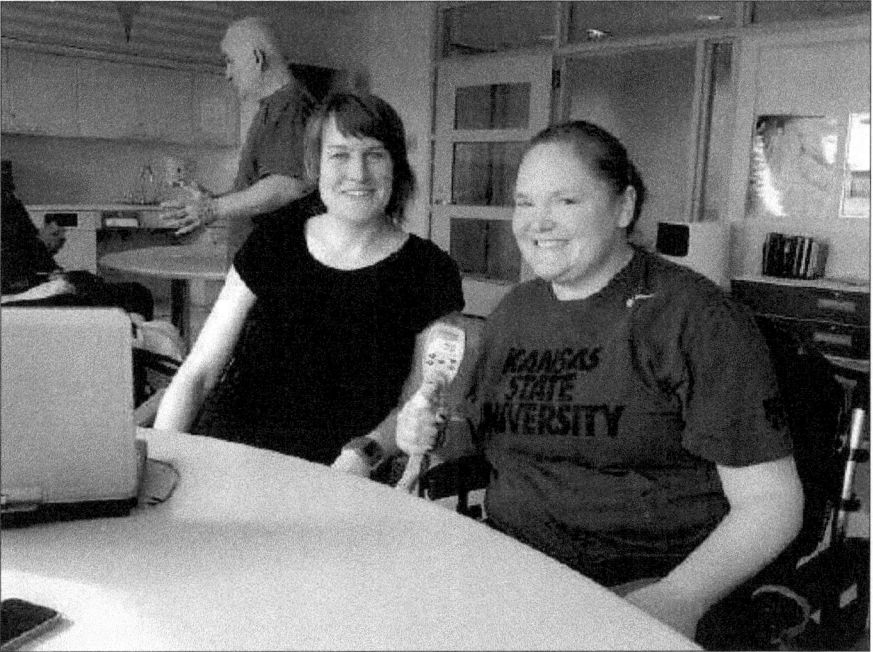

Carrie with occupational therapist, Anne Marie.

Tue, Feb 25, 2014 at 2:49 p.m., from Jeff's email:

Quick Update for Tuesday, February 25th

Carrie has had another good day of therapy, working on tasks like brushing hair, putting on clothes, tying shoes, etc. PTs are also heavily focusing on stretching and mobility now that she's getting stronger and stronger in her trunk and lower body.

Unfortunately, the ENT doc who was supposed to come today was "unfamiliar with granulation issues surrounding tracheas." I'm not a doctor, but what the hell? Isn't that the definition of what an ENT would do? So now we are back to waiting for next week when the original doctor who performed the procedure is supposed to be back in the office. As of Monday she will have been unable to talk for a month.

More soon.

Jeff

Not talking was very difficult for me. Those who know me understand I love to talk, to tell stories, to entertain people. So, when I had to spend one month barely able to communicate verbally it was tough mentally and emotionally. A couple of things lightened that challenge a bit. For one, Jeff and my close friends became adept at lip reading. For another, when I tried to talk, what sounded like a whisper came out, so others could sometimes respond. I got really good at listening during those months. I wish I had some of those keen listening skills today. When people are around someone who can't talk, they often feel they need to fill the void, so they end up talking a lot. I now understand why salespeople and mediators are taught to sit quietly and wait for the other person to speak.

As I've mentioned previously, the ENT doctor missed one of his weekly rounds at RIC because of emergencies elsewhere, and then he was gone for a few weeks on vacation. This meant I hadn't had regular consultations with him, which, as I've noted, was extremely frustrating. So many elements of recovery were going so well, but I worried that missing regular time with an ENT might slow things unnecessarily. A few people suggested that perhaps I needed to seek a second opinion or ask for a new doctor. Jeff and I did discuss that suggestion, me using my non-verbals and Jeff trying to comprehend what I was mouthing. In the end, though, I think we both knew deep down that the ENT we had at Northwestern Memorial Hospital was one of the best, and we needed to stick it out.

As we all discovered at the end of my journey, my windpipe problem was one of the worst—one of that one percent which, unfortunately, did not beat the odds. Time and time again we ended up with the worst-case scenarios with my trachea/

windpipe. Although it was agonizing at times, we survived even my delicate flower of a windpipe trying to rain on our parade.

March 4, 2014

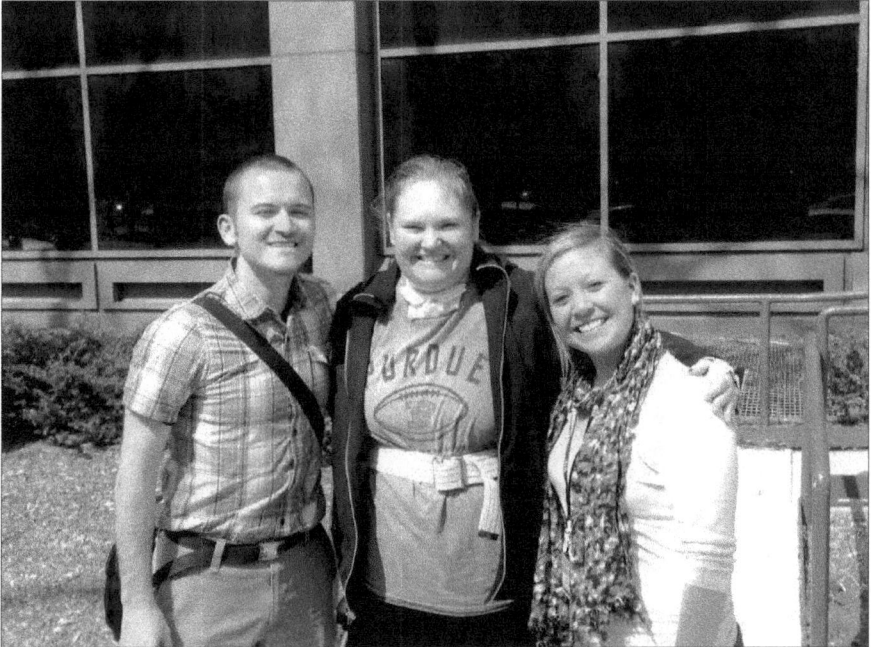

Carrie with physical therapists, Patrick and Jill.
Next page: Carrie walking on the ninth floor.

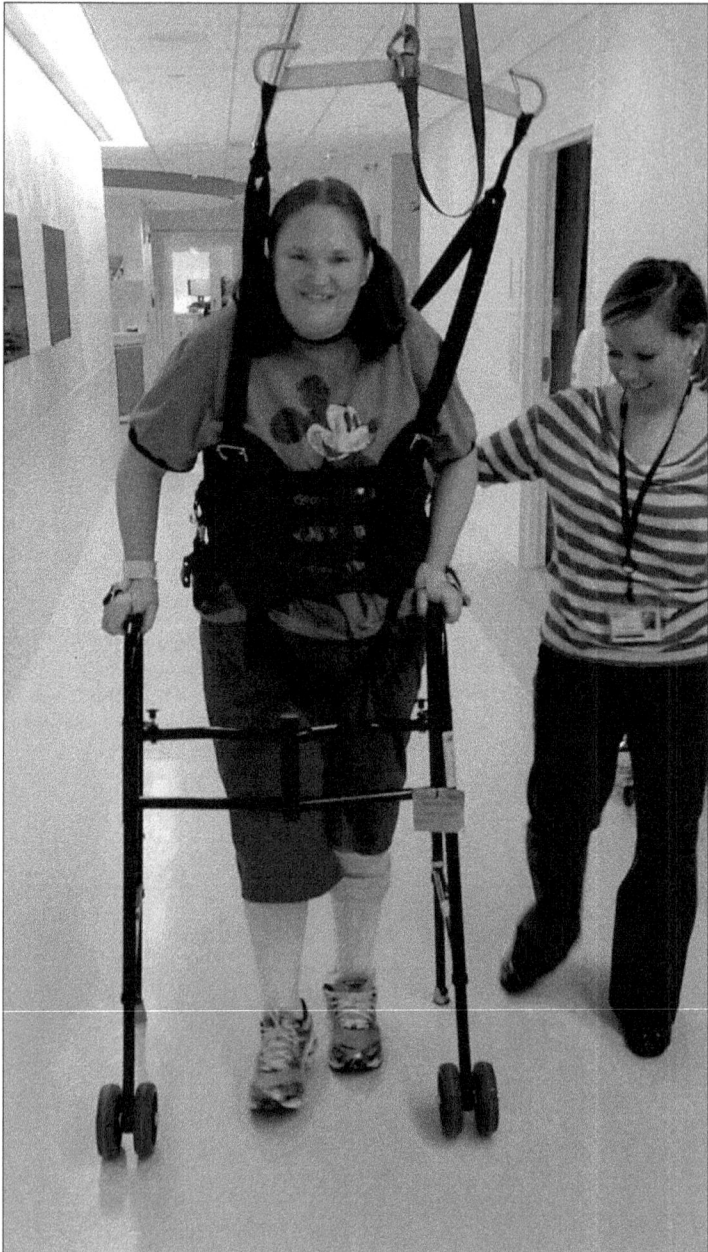

Tue, Mar 4, 2014 at 5:24 P.M., from Jeff's email:

Update for Tuesday, March 4th

Carrie's made yet more great strides toward her recovery this past week. She's gotten up in several walking machines, back on the treadmill for more walking, and yesterday she went up to the ninth floor (the research floor) to walk in an independent harness. She walked around the entire floor supporting her entire body weight one and half times. She told me her therapist had to pick up his jaw from the floor. As I type, they're measuring her for a manual (non-powered) wheelchair. She'll have to do more work to get herself around, but it'll develop better core and upper body strength while her lower body comes back.

On the trach/speech/breathing side, we finally got our appointment with the ENT earlier this afternoon. He answered all of our questions about what our next steps are. He showed Carrie the picture of her original bronchoscopy that clearly showed the narrowing/granulation tissue issue. He told us that he will not go on vacation again, and also that we are scheduled for a 7:30 a.m. procedure tomorrow. He will swap the existing trach tube for a T-tube, which is primarily used as an airway stent, to block the granulation from re-occurring. We were disappointed to hear that the T-tube may be in for up to six months, but are hopeful that after the procedure all speech issues are resolved. She has had zero problems with breathing these past two weeks, so the biggest concern is to get her talking again, but maintain the airway and keep the granulation at bay. The advantage of a T-tube is it will require less suction, since there is an open path to breathe and cough like normal. It is also freestanding due to the design, so does not require the collar and additional maintenance we have now. After the procedure occurs, there is likely to be swelling in the area, so we will be staying at Northwestern for a day or two to be under observation, hopefully returning to RIC Friday or Saturday to get back on the therapy track.

Carrie just returned to her room from PT and told me she stood up all by herself from her chair with zero handrail or therapist assistance. Rock star!

I will try to send more frequent updates over the next few days.

Jeff

Patrick and Jill were always pushing me a bit further in my recovery. I loved that they understood how to motivate me. On the CliftonStrengths assessment from Gallup, my number one strength is competition. That strength played a major role in my recovery. My therapists quickly figured out my motivation came from my competitive spirit, so they pushed me.

I remember vividly the day Patrick said, "Let's go to the ninth floor and walk around." The ninth floor had been renovated to show what the new RIC hospital would look like. It was laid out in a circle, and in the middle of the hallway ceiling was a track to hook up a harness to support someone re-learning to walk. We wheeled my manual wheelchair up there, which took a lot more effort with my arms than merely pushing a joystick! They hooked up the oh-so comfortable harness, then told me on the count of three I would stand. They were there to offer support if I waivered or was off balance.

"One…two…three."

I stood. The majority of my weight was on my legs and it was an odd feeling. After being in a hospital bed for months, a wheelchair, and then being on the treadmill with most of my weight supported by the harness, this was new. My legs felt like spaghetti. My muscles were weak and were not used to this feeling. Patrick told me to go ahead and take a step, so I did. Then another step. Nurses, doctors, other therapists, and patients were milling around the floor saying, "Good job!" or "Keep it up—looking good!" Those were happy words to hear.

After a lap around the hallway, I remember telling Patrick, "I'm tired. I need to rest!" He was happy to let me. As I sat down, he told me how impressed he was. He said he'd had the idea to come up here, but he was not sure I would be able to walk, putting all of my weight on my legs. He said, "You amaze me daily. You are rocking it!" That made my day!

Brooke came to visit that day and got to come see me in action on the ninth floor. Patrick decided just walking was too easy, so he put some objects on the floor that I had to step over. In a normal situation, you would think, "No big deal." Turns out when you have not fully used your muscles for a few weeks, lifting your leg high enough to walk over an object takes a lot of energy and concentration. I did okay, but a bit unstable on my feet. "We'll keep working on it!" Patrick said.

The ENT doctor finally returned from vacation. We had an appointment set up with him and I was going no matter what. I wanted answers. We had to wait in the doctor's office for more than an hour as he had been called into an emergency surgery. I remember Jeff getting frustrated and I told him, "Hey! I would want him to help me if it was an emergency!"

The doctor finally came into the room and apologized for the last few weeks. Within minutes I was no longer angry at him. I remembered why I liked working with him. He understood my frustrations and acknowledged them. He was personable. He talked to us about our son. He recognized we had to figure out how to fix this. We discussed the surgery the next day and that the trachea tube (T-tube) was our best option. We talked through the pros and cons and what other options we may have (stent, etc.) The T-tube seemed to be the best choice. I left his office feeling good that we had a plan. I went back to RIC for a good night's sleep in preparation for an early surgery.

I'm not sure I got great sleep with my not-so-fun roommate. I stayed in our day room as long as possible to avoid her talking my ear off and complaining. I needed only positive influences in my life at this juncture. I was getting better and needed all the energy I had to go towards my recovery, not towards dealing with difficult people. It may sound mean, but I had to be selfish at times to ensure my recovery. I also said "No thank you" at times to people who wanted to visit. It wasn't that I didn't want to see them, but I got tired easily. If I'd had visitors multiple days in a row, I would often tell Jeff (my personal scheduler) that I needed a night off.

March 6, 2014

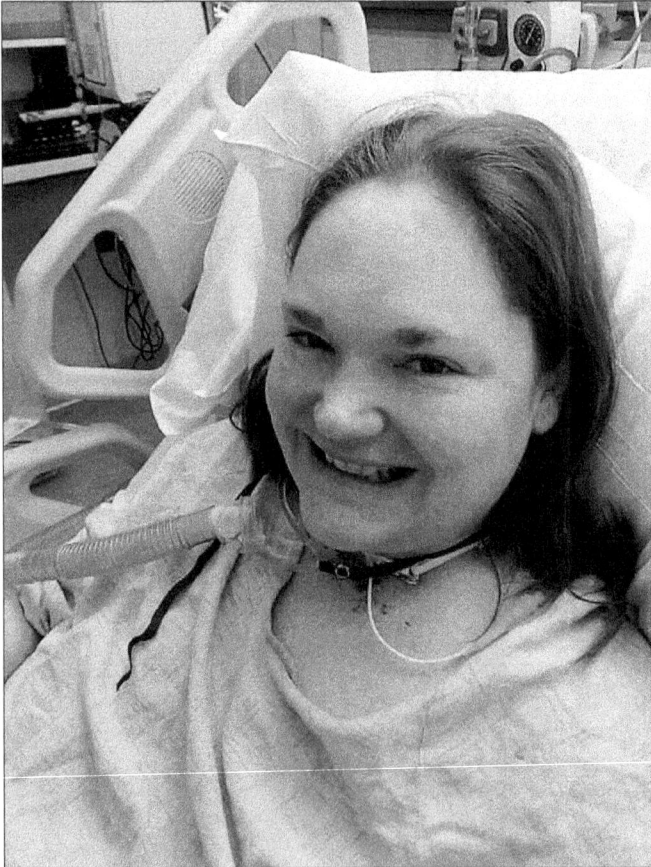

Carrie in hospital bed off the vent!

Thu, Mar 6, 2014 at 9:44 a.m., from Jeff's email:

Update for Thursday, March 6th

Carrie had a long day yesterday. We woke up at 5:30 a.m. to get prepped for our long two-block ride to Northwestern. We arrived at pre-op at 6:45 and then waited until 9:00 to go in. The doctor was able to successfully remove the trach tube and install the t-tube with no issues, in less than thirty minutes. They woke Carrie up and had her talk, but once she started talking, they realized there was more granulation tissue at the lower end of where the trach had been. They put her back under and spent ninety more minutes removing that tissue. She was out of the OR and back in the recovery rooms shortly after noon. She is so happy to be able to talk again! We were stuck in recovery from 12:30 until 9:00 p.m. as there were a whole lot of emergency surgeries that kept usurping ICU rooms. Carrie spent the night in the ICU and, as of this morning, is feeling good and has less pain and swelling. Breathing has been great, and she's ready to get back in the rehab groove. She's waiting to hear from the doctor about removing her peg tube/g-tube while we're there, but the hope is she will go back to RIC this afternoon, rather than staying longer at Northwestern.

Jeff

What a joy it was to speak again. It's difficult to realize how much we rely on talking to communicate our wants and needs.

By this time in my ordeal, I had become used to going into surgery, but this one was a bit different. They actually woke me up mid-surgery. I remember the doctor asking me to talk and me getting excited to talk, then realizing it was not my full voice. I remember looking around at the doctors, anesthesiologists, and nurses. They looked concerned. They asked if they could put me back under anesthesia so they could get some granulation tissue that must be below the new T-tube.

"Yes – please just fix it!"

They put me back to sleep. I remember waking up what seemed like a few minutes later but in actuality was a few hours later. They let Jeff come back to the surgery recovery area so I could show off my voice. The doctor came to see how I was doing. The T-tube seemed to be working. I gave him a big smile and thanked him with my own voice for his help! I also asked him why I still had my feeding tube. They had told me they would remove it in surgery. He explained that it seemed to catch a little bit when he went to pull it out, so he wanted the surgeons to look at it. He said they would come back in the morning to remove it.

It then became a waiting game to get a room for the night. An hour passed, then another. The beds in the surgery recovery area are tiny and uncomfortable. The nurse would come by and apologize that they had not found a room yet. The doctor wanted me to be in an ICU room to closely monitor my breathing for twenty-four hours. We ended up in recovery for more than nine hours due to multiple emergencies which filled the ICU rooms. I told Jeff that although I was annoyed, it was nice not to be the emergency.

When I finally got to the ICU, Jeff got me settled then took off to sleep at our friend's condo. He was exhausted. It felt odd to have a nurse almost constantly checking on me again. In the ICU it was one nurse to every two patients, which is awesome when you need acute care. I felt a little like an imposter being there, appearing so much healthier than most of their patients. I remember thinking how odd the room looked, how different it seemed now that I was fully coherent and could move my body, roll myself over in bed, change the TV channel myself. I did a little happy dance in my bed, careful not to set off one of the million machines or monitors.

The next morning the doctors made their rounds and I was given the green light to head back to RIC. I asked the doctors if I could get my peg tube (feeding tube) pulled out. They said they would see what they could do. So I went on with my morning, getting in the chair, which wasn't easy. At RIC, my PTs had started to use something called a slide board to help me get in and out of bed to the wheelchair or from my wheelchair to the toilet. It looks like a smaller version of a snowboard. They slide it under your bottom and you move your hips side to side and slide onto the chair or toilet. It saves them having to use the big Hoyer lift. In the hospital, I did not have my slide board or my walker to help stabilize me, so getting out of bed was harder. Two nurses helped me stand, somehow shuffle, and pivot to the chair. I made it! I ate breakfast and watched some TV, waiting for someone to tell me if my tube could be taken out and when I could go back to RIC. I was anxious to try to get in some rehab if possible that day. Had to keep moving! Next thing I knew a woman came in and said, "I am here to remove your peg tube!"

I wasn't sure what to expect.

"Ok – let's do this. Can you raise your gown?"

She looked at the tube, tugged a little bit and then said "Ok, brace yourself! This may hurt a bit." And with that she basically put her foot against my chair and literally yanked the tube out. I thought she was going to fly across the room.

I sat there in shock. It hurt like a mother f***ker when she pulled that thing out but then the pain started to dull and I thought to myself, "Hooray, another thing removed from my body!"

The ENT doctor stopped by later on to check in with me. Breathing was fine. I was talking. I was feeling pretty good. He told me I could go back to RIC and get back to therapy. I would see him in six months to get the T-tube removed. No submerging in water, but he said I could get in a pool, which was a huge relief. I missed being in the water. It was going to be hard not diving in during the summer, but I would take whatever I could get.

March 7, 2014

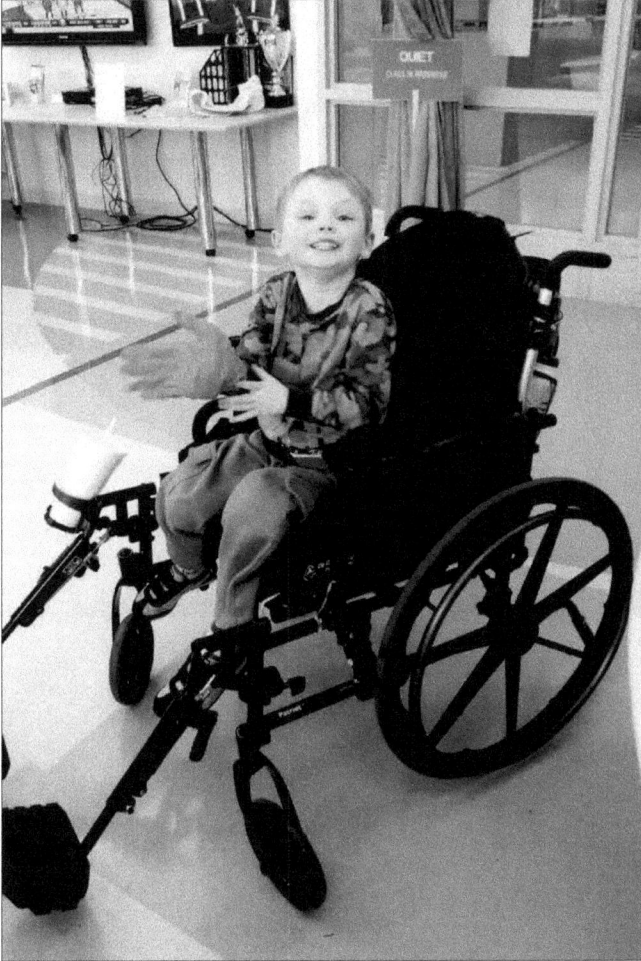

*Will sitting in Mom's wheelchair with
his blue gloves on.*

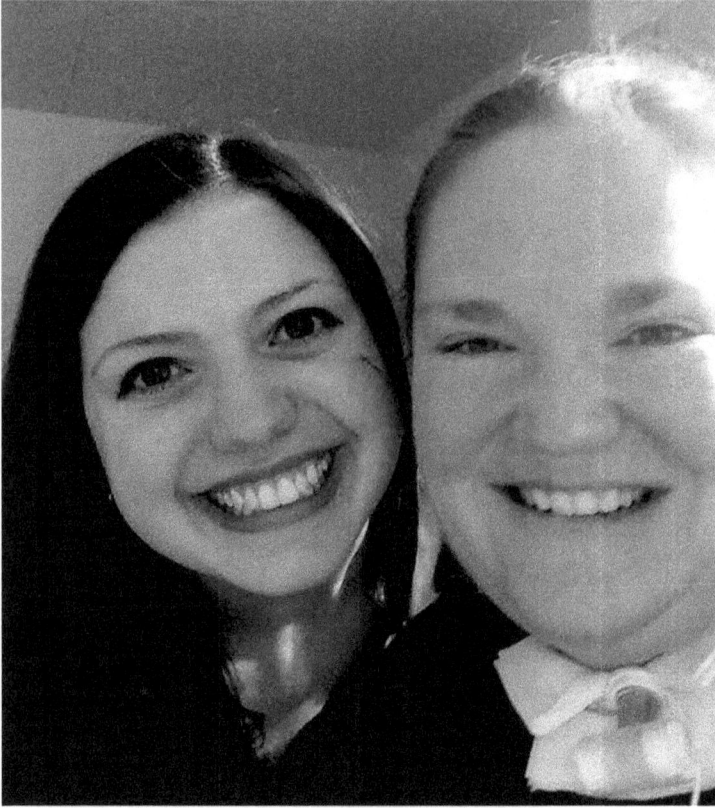

Carrie with occupational therapist Zoe,
who stopped by to visit Carrie during her new job.

Fri, Mar 7, 2014 at 5:17 p.m., from Jeff's email:

Update for Friday, March 7th

Carrie returned to RIC late in the afternoon on Thursday. She's been resting and dealing with a little bit of swelling and pain today, but the good news is she is able to talk!!! There's a period of adjustment with the T-tube obviously, but it'll just go along with all of the other changes that have happened today. She also had her g-tube removed while she was at Northwestern, and had her last IV removed this afternoon. So the only non-standard part remaining is the T-tube, and it'll be capped ninety-nine percent of the time.

Originally Carrie returned too late to get on the therapy schedule, but the floor supervisors got her into speech, OT, and PT sessions today. She officially transferred out of a power chair into a manual chair, did a little walking on the treadmill, and also worked on slide transfers in and out of bed, rather than the lift system.

To go along with all of that, a reorg of the floor due to some incoming patients needing single rooms, meant we have moved rooms yet again. She's now in room 706 with a new roomie.

I had just gotten used to my crazy roommate and enjoying my corner view with windows on two sides when they told me I had to move rooms again. My new roommate was a woman of about sixty years old, who had cancer that had unfortunately resulted in paralysis of her legs. She and her husband were quite cordial, and, I could tell, quite intelligent. She owned her own company, which her son was in the process of taking over. When he visited, I would often excuse myself to give them privacy in discussing business matters. She was the opposite of my old roommate; she went to bed early, was very quiet, and mostly kept to herself. Occasionally at night she would call out and ask me how I was doing. I think she was intrigued by me and my illness and was hopeful she could recover as I was doing.

I was in a manual wheelchair these days, and from the moment I got out of bed and into it, I was usually off for the day. I was getting back to listening to music and I had my headphones on much of the time. If other people were in therapy and I was waiting for mine to start, I'd be sitting there jamming to the latest tunes. Music played a tremendous role in my recovery. It calmed me when I could not sleep and it pumped me up for the exertion of regaining mobility. Music was welcome company when Jeff or my friends couldn't be there with me.

I was sore after they took out the trachea tube. The T-tube felt odd. I was able to talk, but my breathing did not seem totally normal. I remember walking in PT and having to stop because my breathing was labored. We thought it was just my body getting back into shape.

I was pushing myself to do whatever they asked in therapy. Lying in bed in the morning, I was now able to help get my underwear and shorts on. My sports bra was still a tough one, but I was getting better with that as well as my t-shirt. I got better and better at slide transfers, so getting me in and out of bed was much easier. Showers at night also became much more pleasant as I was able to transfer with the slide board. I was working on my ankle strength as they were still so weak and often buckled. But I was giving it my all.

March 12, 2014

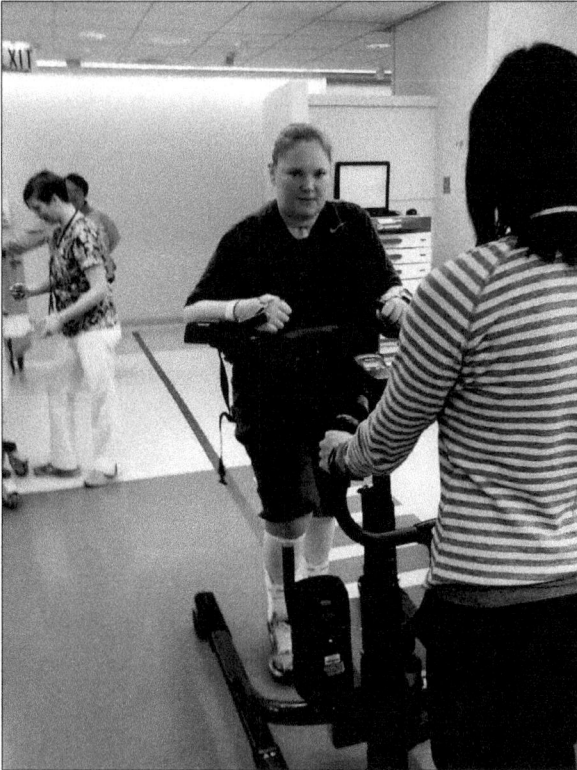

*Carrie walking around her floor with a machine
helping her balance.*

Wed, Mar 12, 2014 at 2:21 p.m. from Jeff's email:

Update for Wednesday, March 12th

Carrie has had a good week. She's loved being able to talk to all her nurses, doctors and therapists. She's picked up a LOT of gossip on the floor as well, so she's in her element! At Carrie's request, today we talked to the ENT doctor as a follow-up from last week's procedure. He performed a quick scope of the T-tube and noticed a little bit of granulation tissue below where the old trach was. He decided he wants Carrie to come back in tomorrow (Thursday) for another (and we hope final) procedure. If he sees no additional granulation above where the trach was, he'll clean up the lower area and just remove the T-tube, as Carrie's airway is obviously very susceptible to granulation around foreign objects. If there is granulation on the upper portion of the T-tube he'll clean it all up and replace the T-tube.

We're obviously hoping for the first option— cleanup and removal of the tube entirely to let her airway heal up. We don't know the exact time for the procedure, but we'll probably be there all day tomorrow. If it's just a clean and replace we'll be back at RIC Friday, but if the tube is removed, they'll probably keep her over the weekend to come back to RIC on Monday.

On to the good reports! Carrie has transitioned to a manual wheelchair! No more power wheels for her, she's got to use her own muscle to get around. She was also able to fully dress herself and get out of bed into her new chair in one-third the time the therapist had allotted. This included tying her shoes! She's also been making great progress on the walking front— using a walker, supporting her full body weight, harnessed only for safety. She's been a little more tired this week than in the past.

We appreciate all of the continued support, cards, flowers and visits. I'll send another update soon.

Jeff

I was so glad we had the ENT doctor check me out that day he was doing rounds at RIC. I had told my RIC doctor that things just did not feel right. I have to say one benefit of having Guillain-Barré is that I came to know my body extremely well. I now know to pay attention when something doesn't feel right, to go with my gut, and be my own advocate. I cannot stress that enough to loved ones and caretakers of friends. If the patient cannot fully talk or communicate for themselves, PLEASE be their advocate. Doctors, nurses, everyone, all want to help patients, but they don't always pick up on the subtle clues or signs that a family member or the patient notices. SPEAK UP in a constructive manner. It doesn't help to yell, scream, or treat any of the staff poorly. They want to help you, but if they are busy, you must get their attention and ask for assistance. You can be polite and be an advocate at the same time.

I was rocking that manual wheelchair, but wow did it wear me out. Turns out those PT folks were smart when they made me change over from the electric chair to the manual. I went from doing laps around the halls to making maybe two laps a day. My arms were out of shape! It felt good to be using my muscles again though.

It was so energizing to be able to talk to all my therapists, nurses, PCTs, doctors—to be able to ask my own questions, to tell them when it hurt, to tell them when I was happy, and to share secrets with the staff about my old roommate. I also asked them for the latest and greatest gossip. I was beginning to feel like my old self. Socializing, meeting other patients, getting to express who I really was. I cannot explain how hard that is to do when you cannot speak.

March 18, 2014

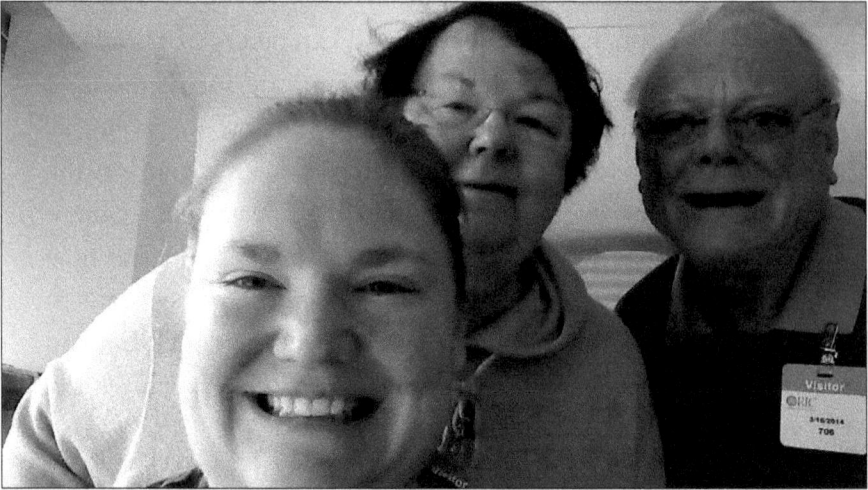

Carrie and her parents in the rehab hospital.

Tue, Mar 18, 2014 at 5:12 p.m., from Jeff's email:

Update for Tuesday, March 18th

Carrie's procedure last week went so so. The good news is, we were only in recovery for a couple of hours, and then spent another night in the ICU before returning to RIC. The bad news is, the doctor saw more granulation on the lower portion of the trachea where her tube was originally, so her delicate flower of a windpipe needs more time to heal. The ENT also wants to replace the existing T-tube with a custom length tube that will hopefully 'stent' more of the airway open and keep that tissue from regrowing, to let the whole area stabilize and heal. We've now asked the ENT for a "buy three procedures, get the fourth for free" as we'll have at least two more in our future.

Carrie has been making great "strides" with her standing and walking work. She's been up and down in several different machines. She's completely abandoned slide boards for the much easier stand and pivot with a support walker. Yesterday she made two laps around the floor with just the walker (no harness, no helping hands). Dick and Kathy spent the weekend with Carrie, which was great for everyone involved– the Campbells got to spend time together and I got some more sleep at home. Dick's new nickname is "the paparazzi" as he was in charge of taking pics and videos on his phone. I'm sure by now everyone in Lincoln has seen every second of video footage.

Today, Carrie got to attend the community re-entry group, which takes a group of patients out for lunch and an activity. Today's outing was to Lucky Strike bowling alley where we enjoyed some burgers and knocked down some pins. Carrie split time throwing the ball from her wheelchair and a few frames standing with the walker and throwing. Ever a competitor, she was disappointed in her score, but pointed out she didn't come in last.

Many of you have asked when Carrie will be discharged from RIC and be back home. Her therapy team hopes to keep her approximately another four to six weeks, but we do not yet have a set date. We're still hoping to conquer the goals of walking unassisted and going up and down stairs, to avoid major home modification work. Our best guess is sometime mid to late April.

I was so bummed when I woke up and found out that I still had a T-tube in my throat. On top of that, the doctor and Jeff had to break the news to me that I had at least a couple more surgeries ahead of me because the granulation tissue had grown below the T-tube. I learned a lot during my GBS journey and one of those lessons was that even when you think you cannot take one more piece of bad news, deep down inside you find a way. I think about half of my strength came from within and the other half from my friends and family, especially Jeff. I remember weeping in recovery when Jeff told me the disappointing news. And I remember him being strong, rubbing my hand, and arm over and over again and telling me we would get through it.

I kept questioning if this nightmare was ever going to end. I remember asking if I would ever get to swim again. I love to swim. I love to be in the water. Swimming was one of my favorite workouts. Whenever I was in a bad place or hurting, I took the advice of Kent Seacrest, my friend who'd had GBS, and I went to my happy place. My happy place was my parent's pool, a clear blue sky, warm bright sun, and me swimming gracefully and peacefully through the cool brisk water. Up and down in the water, free to dive under, jump up, and feel the water on my face, neck, and hair. I started doubting I would ever get to enjoy going under water again.

With Jeff's help I found strength. I returned to RIC determined to keep pushing myself so I could walk independently and eventually conquer those stairs. It was such an uplift to have my parents visit that weekend and for me to show them how far I had come since I'd last seen them. I think it is probably what little kids feel when they finally learn to walk. They have their entire family cheering them on and they are so proud to see their parents so proud of them. Jeff did not exaggerate when he said my dad was the paparazzi. It was like he was capturing his child's first steps, and in a way, it was just as monumental. Before GBS, I took for granted getting up from bed in the morning, walking to the bathroom, taking a shower. The easiest things were now so hard and took so much strength and energy. I look back and I am proud that I don't take those daily activities for granted any longer.

I thought it was so cool that the RIC took patients on outings to help them re-acclimate into society. It was one thing to wheel my chair through the halls of the hospital where the floors are level and easy to maneuver. It was an ordeal to try to wheel my chair along Chicago sidewalks in March when it was thirty-five degrees and the wind was blowing in my face. There seemed to be construction on both sides of the street at each turn. And even though Chicago seems flat, I swear that every sidewalk seemed to be uphill. On our bowling trip, I pushed myself for a few blocks but was quickly falling behind, so Jeff was nice enough to help push me to the bowling alley.

Real food! Even though my appetite wasn't fully back, it was a treat to escape hospital food! I love bowling. When I was a kid my mom bowled in a Thursday morning league, so she would take me to the bowling alley day care to play with my friends. After my mom was done bowling, we would eat lunch at the restaurant across the street called the Pantry where I would order this fun kids drink called a "green river." Or we would eat at the bowling alley's restaurant, Fred and Ruby's— best hamburger in Lincoln. In high school I went bowling every night with my friends, through a program called "Keep kids off drugs – go bowling!" We would meet at the bowling alley, bowl our free game, then go out and do stupid kid stuff.

Bowling is just one of those activities that brings back great memories for me, so I was excited to hear that my outing was to the bowling alley.

Now as you have learned I am a very competitive person. I don't like losing. Obviously, I wasn't in tip-top bowling shape so I had to swallow my pride and be happy with my score of forty-seven. I threw some of the balls sitting in my wheelchair which was extremely hard. I had to throw the ball on the side of the wheelchair at an awkward angle. I also stood a few times and threw the ball, using a ramp that helped guide it. I now realize that ramp is used for kids who can't lift and throw the ball. I underestimated how hard it would be to keep my balance on my unsteady legs, pick up a bowling ball weighing only six pounds, then throw it down a lane. Given those challenges, I was thrilled to hit some pins!

March 24, 2014

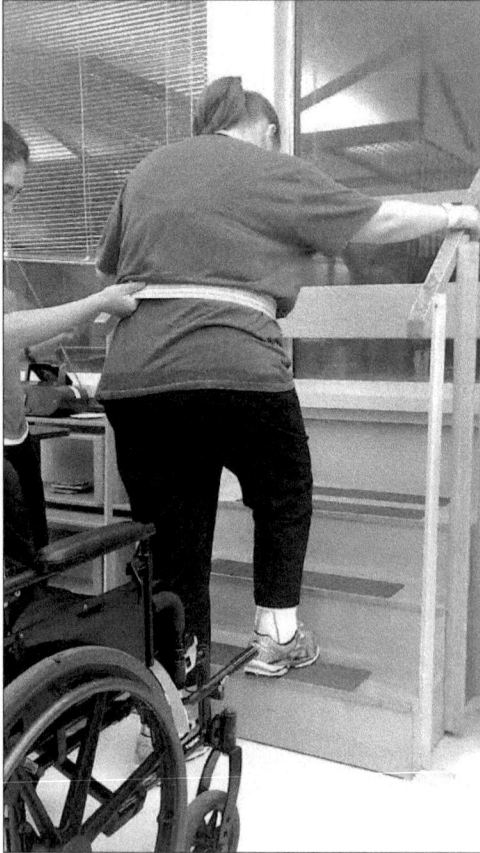

*Carrie working on stairs so she can
go home!*

186

Mon, Mar 24, 2014 at 9:44 AM, from Jeff's email:

Update for Monday, March 24th

The last few days have been a little rough. Wednesday morning Carrie was struggling a little bit to breathe so the decision was made to take her to the ER at Northwestern. The ENT doc came right down between surgeries and took a look through a scope at her T-tube. He saw a lot of granulation tissue—more than he expected. So we ended up having a trach tube reinserted later in the day on Wednesday. To top that off, while we were in the post-op recovery room, her attending physician from RIC came over and told us her insurance was denying readmittance to rehab. So after about a million phone calls and emails and text messages, we spent the night at Northwestern and were readmitted to RIC late in the afternoon on Thursday. Friday, Saturday and Sunday were full of therapies—very focused on preparing to go home. She's been working hard on stairs, car transfers, and getting stronger at standing and walking.

As of now, we are only guaranteed through today at RIC, approval pending every week from the insurance company. Our therapists and case manager have been on top of things, getting us prepped for full-day therapy at an outpatient facility, as well as ordering the things we'll need until she "graduates": a hospital bed, temporary wheelchair, walker, etc. Our therapists are hoping for two more weeks with a tentative discharge date of April 7th, but things should be ready here at home by mid-week if we have to make the move. The biggest stumbling block right now is the breathing. We're still waiting on the custom T-tube to arrive, and once that's swapped in, we'll probably spend at least a day or two in the ICU waiting to see if the granulation keeps occurring. Then she'll probably have the custom tube in for six to eight months unless the ENT feels the issue resolves sooner. We're definitely hoping for sooner. On a positive note, the ENT did say she could get into a pool with the T-tube, just not actually submerge or swim. So that's a small positive!

More fun with my trachea. I went on the RIC patient outing on Tuesday and felt good, but once I got home, I started feeling not so great. I remember telling my respiratory therapist before bedtime that I felt off and that my breathing did not seem normal. I had to listen to my body when it was telling me something was not right. So many times, though, I doubted what I was feeling and figured I was just making a big deal out of nothing. That must be the "Nebraska nice" in me. I never wanted to bother people—nurses, doctors, or my family—more than I was already doing. I eventually learned I had to listen to my body because it was always right!

I did not sleep well, and I asked for a breathing treatment to clear out my T-tube in the middle of the night. It was harder to breathe after the treatment which was rare.

"Something is wrong. I'm having trouble breathing," I told Jeff as soon as he showed up the next morning. He got the nurse, and everyone went into overdrive. As you would expect, when a patient says they can't breathe, people take it seriously. Within twenty minutes I was in an ambulance on my way to Northwestern Memorial Hospital.

The ENT came down between his surgeries, took one look and shook his head. He told me that the granulation tissue had grown extremely quickly below the T-tube and that he was going to have to put my trach back in to keep my airway open until the custom T-tube arrived. The trach meant that my speech would go away again. You can imagine how well I took that news. I was devastated. The situation just seemed to keep going from bad to horrible.

Things were about to get more interesting. After being in the ER for a few hours while the doctor took care of an emergency case (mine was serious but I was stable and they were giving me extra oxygen through my nose), they then took me up to surgery to put in the trach. I woke up in recovery late that afternoon. I was back to not talking, so Jeff read my lips. I was down and bummed but happy to be breathing normally again. I was just starting to feel a little better when the ENT doctor and my doctor from RIC walked into my room. Something was up.

"We have some tough news," my RIC doctor said. "Your insurance is denying your return to RIC. They think you are able to go home."

Tears immediately welled up in my eyes.

"I think we need to keep you overnight here for observation," the ENT doctor said, then he winked. "We will find you a room and that will also give us time to figure out the insurance issue."

My head started reeling. It was too soon! I was making such good progress but was not quite there yet. I could walk a bit but had not tried stairs yet. I could not fully transfer to the bathroom myself. I was not ready and my team at RIC agreed.

Immediately Jeff got on the phone with our insurance company, the HR person at my work, and RIC. Jeff was also freaking out. We didn't have a ramp at home. There are stairs to both our garage and front doors. How would we manage? I am not a dainty girl; they could not lift me into the house.

I got a room on a non-ICU floor since the doctor felt I was stable. That was good for Jeff because the pull-out beds were more comfortable than the chairs in the ICU room. We should go back and count the number of nights Jeff slept in the hospital. And the poor guy has a bad back. Did I mention he wins husband of the year for the next decade? We went to bed unsure of what would happen the next day. I still had not been cleared to go back to RIC.

The next morning Jeff went back to making phone calls. By early afternoon, we were headed back to RIC. We owe a huge thanks to a number of people who worked to make that possible. So the ambulance came to get me. The two-block transfer cost more than $1000. I know that because a few of the trips ended up being coded as "non-emergency" and guess whose health care does not cover non-emergency ambulance transfers? Once I got home and saw the bills, I ended up spending hours and hours getting doctor's letters to submit to our health insurance. The doctors had to verify that there was no other way to transfer me since I was on a vent. I am proud to say I won that battle!

I arrived "home" at RIC late afternoon so I had missed therapy for the day. I was disappointed and very motivated to get going on the hard stuff: stairs! I went back to my room, got in my wheelchair and did laps around the halls because I was anxious to get my strength back. Then on the transfer, I told the nurses, "I can do it!" and worked on standing and pivoting back into bed.

I remember during this time reflecting how far I had come. I went from lying in bed twenty-four hours a day and feeling just horrifically awful to doing laps around the rehab hospital floor and having to be told I had to go back to my room for bed. I was already counting my blessings and I was not yet able to walk. The prognosis had not been good, and I was proving those doctors wrong. I still had a long way to go to get back to my old self, but my progress was worth celebrating! I took full advantage of the upcoming days in therapy. I knew my time at RIC was limited, and I was going to be going home any day.

Brooke came to visit me that Friday night. I had therapy scheduled that evening at five, which was rare on a Friday, but I was not complaining. A new PT from another floor was assigned to me. She asked if I wanted to go to another floor and practice stairs. YES, I did! I walked up my first set of stairs that night and would practice any chance they gave me. I also came back down to my floor and walked down the hallway with my walker for twenty feet. I was so pumped and proud of myself. And Brooke caught it all on camera for Jeff and my parents!

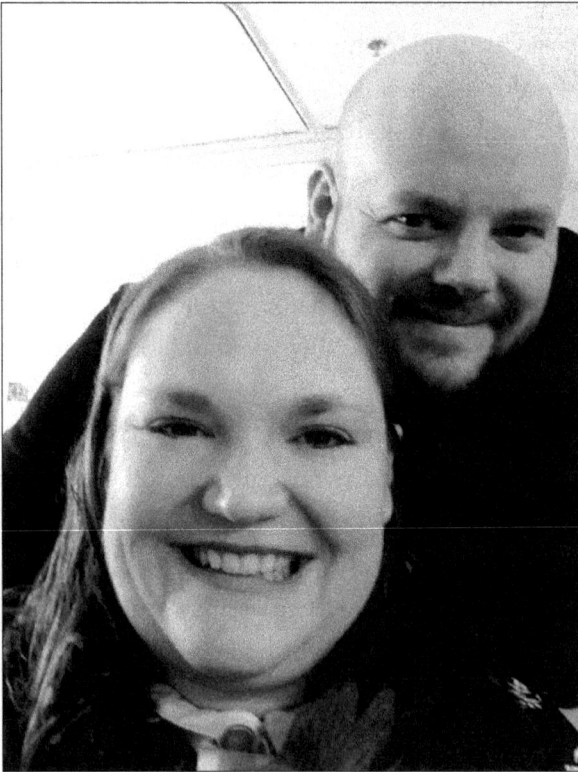

Carrie and Jeff before first date night, breaking free of rehab hospital!

April 2, 2014

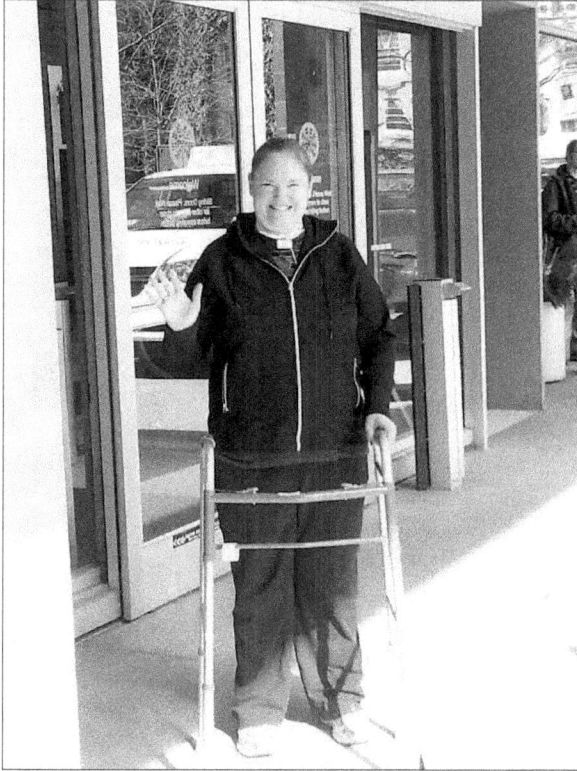

*Carrie successfully meets her goal to walk
out of the Rehab hospital.*

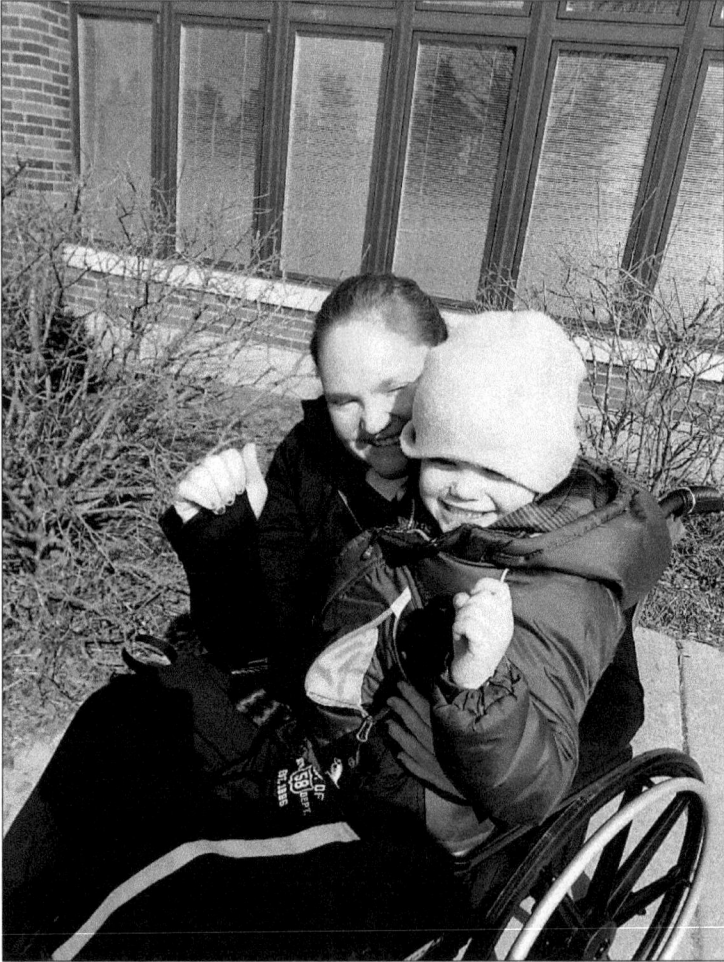

April 2, 2014
Carrie picks up Will at childcare and tells him she is home!

Wed, Apr 2, 2014 at 8:37 p.m., from Jeff's email:

Update for Wednesday April 2nd

Lots of ups and downs over the last long week, but the first and foremost information to impart is that we are officially discharged from RIC and now at home. Carrie's original goal was to walk out of the rehab hospital, and she accomplished that today. Being home has already proven to not be without its challenges, but Carrie is determined to get into a new routine here. She walked up the temporary ramp we installed to the front door, and also made it up the stairs inside to sleep in her own bed tonight. Guess we won't need the hospital bed! We start outpatient full-day rehab at a facility in Wheeling, Illinois on Friday. This is Monday-Friday full-day therapy: speech, occupational and physical therapists will work her over and get her going on new routines.

On an ENT note, we had a slight setback last week as we were told the custom T-tube was going to be delayed until April 18th, but found out yesterday that it was expedited and will be shipped this coming Monday. The ENT doctor came to see Carrie yesterday at RIC and said he would schedule us for the replacement T-tube procedure Wednesday. So we'll have a good start on outpatient therapy, but then spend a few days back at Northwestern to ensure all is well after the replacement.

Jeff

I am not sure what kind of omen it was, but the ride home proved to be more eventful than I would have liked. We were driving home from the hospital and Jeff took the turn to stay on I-94 while some traffic goes straight onto Hwy 41. Two right lanes curve off to continue on I-94 and we were in the left of the two lanes. A woman in the right lane decided she did not want to stay on I-94 and tried to cross three lanes of traffic including cutting right in front of us! She clipped the front ride side of our car where I was sitting. I remember the accident in slow motion. I screamed. The woman's car knocked us into the median between I-94 and Hwy 41. Cars going eighty miles per hour whizzed past us on both sides. I didn't move. I remember praying I was all right.

"I don't want to go back to the hospital!" I said to Jeff, tears running down my face.

Jeff quickly leaned over to inspect me. I was ok! My arm that had been resting on the car door was a little sore, but that was it. We didn't dare get out of our cars due to the high volume of traffic. We called 911 and asked them to send a police officer. It took forty-five minutes for the officer to come. I could not believe our rotten luck that day. All I wanted to do was go home. The officer came, took pictures, took our accounts of the accident, and we were finally on our way. At least we could drive our car. The other car had to be towed.

Poor Jeff. This ended up being a huge nightmare for him. We had to get a rental car, work with the insurance agency, and eventually testify in arbitration as the other driver sued us, claiming we ran into her. People these days! They tried to trip Jeff up in court talking about how I had just gotten out of the hospital and that he must have been distracted. It still makes me mad to think someone would lie about trying to cut across traffic. We could have been seriously injured. But we were okay, our car got fixed, and our insurance agency won the lawsuit!

After the hubbub of the car accident, we went home so I could get something to eat and rest a bit before going to surprise Will at childcare! I was so excited to pick him up.

"Mom!" he shouted, visibly excited to see me.

I got hugs from all of his teachers who had been second moms to him while I was in the hospital. It was so amazing how many people made such a huge difference in our lives while I was recovering! I am so grateful Will had such a great support system.

We headed home and Will was super pumped to see me walk up the ramp. He got his bike out and rode up and down the ramp, of course trying to go up with Mommy. Three-year-olds can't quite grasp the safety issues with that. It felt like life was back to normal!

I also was pretty darn proud that I had walked out of RIC that day with my walker. It was a bittersweet moment. It was exciting to be leaving and going home, but also very scary. I had come to rely on the nurses, PCTs, and care team for so much. The rooms, hallways, and therapy are all designed to support someone in a wheelchair, with a walker, or other mobility assistance device. I didn't realize how handy that was until I went home or visited somewhere and realized the world is not built for someone in a wheelchair.

Our bedroom is upstairs, so Jeff had rented a hospital bed and put it up in the playroom/den on our first floor. We have only a half bath on the main floor so if I wanted a shower (I badly wanted to shower in my own house), I had to make it up the stairs. I told Jeff I was going to climb those stairs, but just once a day. So after dinner, playing with Will, and reading books, I slowly climbed up the steps with Jeff's support. I made it!

Next, we had to tackle the shower. My legs were still not fully healed, and my balance was still way off. I had just started using the walker and had been in my wheelchair up until that day I left RIC. I needed a lot of help to use the walker to get to the shower, then in the shower. Luckily our shower had a bench in it. Jeff would help me get seated and I would shower sitting down. When I was done, Jeff would turn off the shower, put a towel under my feet, and another under the walker. I am proud to say we were successful showering that way for a few weeks. Only once did I slip slightly and start to fall backwards. I was strong enough to hold myself on the bench until Jeff could help me. Another example of how you don't realize how essential muscles are and how much we rely on them for daily tasks.

Jeff also had grab bars installed in all of our bathrooms to help me stand up. These were so helpful, especially at night. (I think our parents are happy we installed them as well for when they visit!)

I started outpatient rehab Friday, a day after getting home. It was good to start on a Friday to learn the ropes of how that center worked. I was scared and nervous about a new routine. Jeff took me the first few days but eventually a car service picked me and two other patients up and drove us to therapy about thirty minutes from our house. This was a huge help to Jeff, and it gave me a chance to meet some new people. On those rides, I learned about new restaurants to try in the area, heard the stories of the other patients, and sometimes I just took a little cat nap.

April 9, 2014

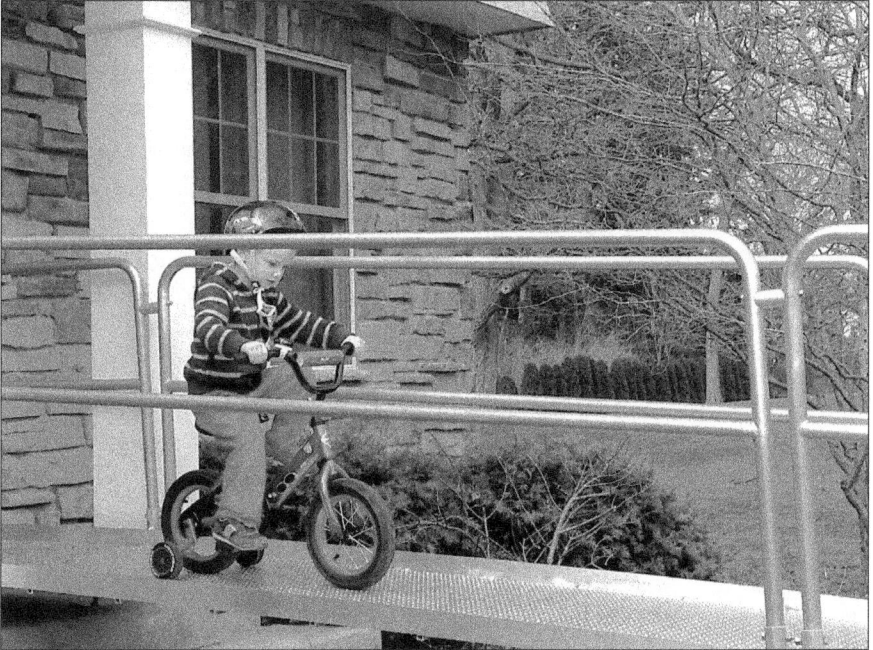

Will riding down the ramp Jeff had installed for Carrie
to get into the house.

Wed, Apr 9, 2014 at 12:53 p.m., from Jeff's email:

Update for Wednesday, April 9th

The past week has been another great week of progress. After relaxing a bit on Thursday, Carrie began full-day outpatient therapy at the RIC facility in Wheeling, Illinois. She had speech, OT and PT for two hours each and was very glad to come home and rest on the couch. We had several visitors over the weekend, and she loved seeing folks, as well as eating some home-cooked meals! Monday and Tuesday, we continued full-day rehab with a heavy focus on getting stronger walking and moving, along with some initial occupational preparation for hopefully getting back to work in late May or early June.

Today we came back down to Northwestern for the custom T-tube replacement procedure. Carrie is out of surgery, awake and TALKING! This tube will probably be in for around six months, but may come out sooner depending on her delicate flower of a windpipe. Our ENT doc will keep us overnight and we'll go home to rest up sometime tomorrow (Thursday). We'll be keeping a close eye on the breathing and coughing but the idea is to keep the tube closed all the time and let her natural breathing path work its magic. We'll take an extra rest day on Friday and hit therapy hard on Monday.

Many folks have already brought us some wonderful meals over the last week, and Carrie's said many more have asked if there's anything we need. Meals and visits are the best things we could ask for right now and Carrie being Carrie has already setup a website to help organize and schedule meal deliveries.

Will is very glad to have Mommy at home, but will now be disappointed that she can call him out for being naughty.

Jeff

I was so excited to have my voice back! As Jeff said, I think Will quite enjoyed when I couldn't yell at him! I felt like I was an old pro at the trachea surgeries. It felt so odd to be back in the ICU where the long tough days in December had started, but to be doing so much better. I could get in and out of bed with the walker and help. I could talk, and I was not in extreme pain. There were moments when I would have flashbacks of the ICU in December and it looked so different. Granted, I was hallucinating back then, and was quite out of it, but the ICU seemed like a different place. I almost felt guilty being in the ICU after getting the T-tube, but I know I needed to be under close watch in in case my windpipe decided to freak out and something went awry. The nurses were amazing and always took excellent care of me, no matter my situation. Nurses are very extraordinary people. I have a special place in my heart for all who cared for me.

April 21, 2014

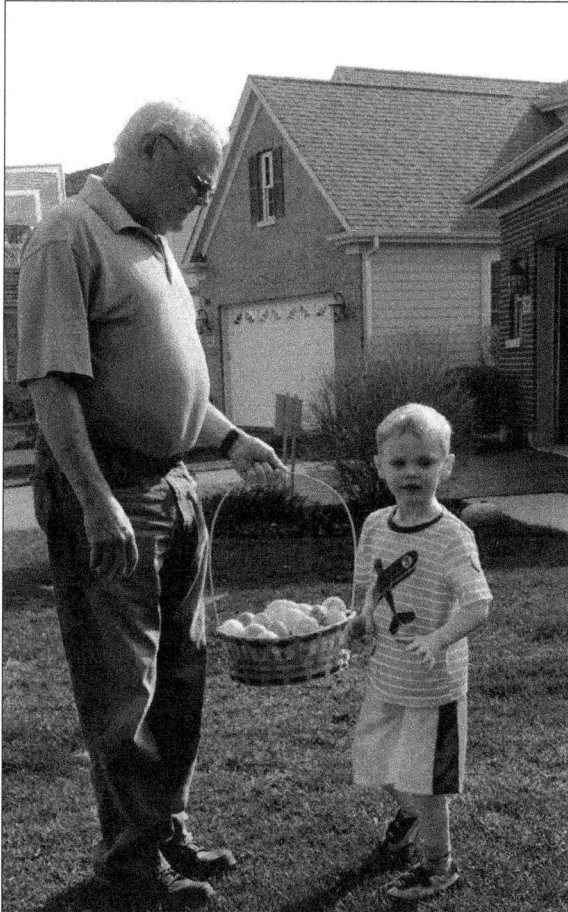

Will and Dick (Carrie's Dad) on Easter 2014.

Mon, Apr 21, 2014 at 5:13 p.m., from Carrie's email:

Jeff has passed the reins to me to write the update emails! He said that it is good occupational therapy for me since one of my OT goals is to get back to lightning-speed typing as I continue to prepare to go back to work.

It was a fantastic Easter here! We were sad to say goodbye to Greg and Ardie (Jeff's parents) who had been helping us out since late January. They were amazing and Will was sad to see his playmates go. My parents and brother Andy arrived on Good Friday. I had the opportunity to go to church on Easter which was wonderful so I could thank God in person for all the blessings he has given us the past few months. It was a beautiful day here so we spent the afternoon outside with an Easter egg hunt for Will, while Dick and Andy told Jeff and me what we should do to our yard.

Great news regarding my delicate flower of a windpipe; the custom T-tube put in April 9th is doing the trick to keep that granulation tissue from growing. Hooray! I have not had any breathing issues and have had to do little suctioning (which is just as fun as it sounds!). We had a follow-up with the ENT today and he scoped my trachea and confirmed no granulation tissue was growing. He said, "Give me a ring in six months and I will take that T-tube out and the hole should close up and we will put this behind us!"

We also had a follow-up with my primary care physician whom I had previously met one time. Since we'd moved, I had just transferred to a new PCP closer to our home right before I got sick. After we went through the events of the last four months, my doctor said, "Wow, I cannot believe what you are telling me. This is by far the worst case of GBS I have ever heard of!" I told him I don't do things half-way!

He was complimentary on my progress based on the last few months!

All-day rehab is definitely paying off. I have kicked the walker to the curb (or I guess set it aside). I was wearing ankle air casts when I left the rehab hospital. I had to wear them all day to help me walk because my ankles were very weak. After countless hours of ankle therapy, I have also gotten rid of those. Once I could talk, I went to one hour of speech and they graduated me from speech! So now I get to have physical therapy (lower body work) and occupational therapy (upper body and fine motor skills), each three hours a day. After six hours, I am tired and hungry when I return home!

I take transportation services to rehab now which saves Jeff or a family member the two hours back and forth. Next week at rehab I see the doctor to discuss a plan to get back to driving and a vocational therapist who will work with me on a plan to return to work. With GBS, my stamina is going to be one of the biggest hurdles for going back to work. I will have to start part time and work up to full time.

It has been so wonderful to be home. It has forced me to stretch myself a bit on bending down to pick something up or work on my standing tolerance while doing the dishes. Will announced last week that the best part of Mommy getting better is she can talk...except when she puts me in timeout!

I hope you each had a wonderful Easter with your family. We would still love to see any of you who live close! We have appreciated the meals people have brought us!

Hugs to all,

Carrie and Jeff

I could not have been more relieved to get those ankle braces off. It made showering so much easier. Before, I had to wear the ankle braces into the shower, get seated and then have Jeff help take them off before we turned on the water. Did I mention I married a saint? I doubt he thought he would see his wife naked wearing ankle casts when he said, "I do."

I remember all the exercises they made me do at rehab to strengthen my ankles. One set of activities involved parallel bars and walking up and down on various types of materials: foam boards, balance beams, etc. I had the parallel bars to help me out if I felt like I was starting to fall. I felt like I was in the Olympics! My favorite activity was using the putting green. The PTs would break it out at the end of our session. I would stand on the foam material and try to putt as many golf balls in the hole as I could. You can imagine I turned it into a huge competition. I held the record for many months until my second-to-last day at therapy when some new guy beat me. It was a good run!

I started to get into a groove at outpatient therapy. To work on my hand coordination in preparation for going back to work, I had to do typing. I still had a bit of pain in my hands at times and they ached when I practiced typing. The funny thing, though, is that I am a pretty fast typist. When I took the skill tests to get a baseline, I was already faster than the speed needed to "pass" that phase of therapy. Since I still had some soreness and pain, they let me continue. I think I set some records for fastest typing by a patient (not that I am competitive or anything).

Going to church on Easter was special to me. I am a religious person, but don't share it very broadly with a lot of people as I view it as personal. I prayed a lot to God while I was sick. I believed God was on my journey with me. Don't get me wrong; I was angry at Him very early on, but I knew He was only giving me as much as I could handle. I believe that. I know there were so many people also praying for me during my illness. People I know really well like my previous church family in Nebraska and lots of friends and relatives. There were also people that I didn't know praying for me. Friends of friends would put me on prayer chains. It all contributed to me getting better. I believe all those prayers lifted me up in tough times and were a part of my healing. I still thank God for how far I have come and for regaining my health.

May 9, 2014

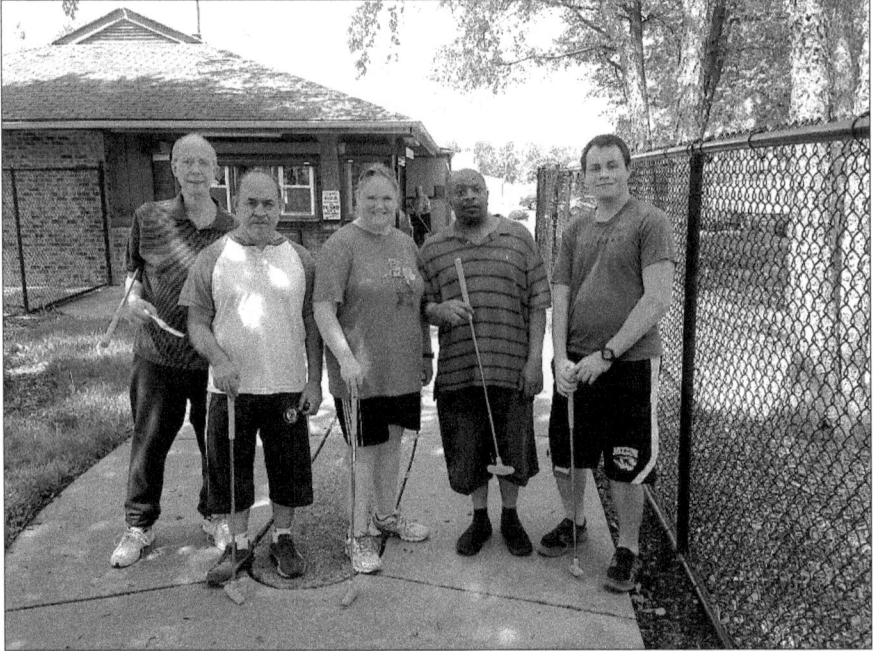

Mini golf therapy with Carrie's outpatient rehab buddies.

Fri, May 9th, 2014 at 3:27 p.m., from Carrie's email:

Hi friends!

I thought I would send out a quick update on my progress as I have been getting some questions on how I am doing. We are getting back to the routines of life!

Therapy has been going great! I have been going about four times a week. I have taken a few Fridays to hang out with Will. My therapists said that was A-OK because I was making such great progress! It was very special going to the Mother's Day brunch with Will and my mom this morning, and last Friday we had a Will and Mommy day (plus grandma Mimi our chauffeur)!

In PT I have been working hard on regaining strength in my legs. My feet are still pretty numb. I tell people it feels like I have ski boots on and every time I step my foot tingles like when it's asleep. I am getting faster and more stable at walking. Will tells me I am not fast enough yet though. He is constantly saying, "Faster, Mommy!" I can see progress though. Last week I did this PT test called the six-minute walk. Basically you walk as fast as you can (safely) and see how far you can walk in six minutes. In the month I have been in outpatient therapy I doubled my distance! Yesterday they asked me what percent I am at with getting back to my old self. I answered sixty-five to seventy percent. They asked what makes up that thirty percent, I said, "Well, I used to run." and I cannot do that yet. The PT said, "Let's go try it!" So I ran down the hallway with a harness machine attached in case I tripped or fell. My feet clomped on the floor due to my numbness but I was running!

In OT, we continue to work on my core strength. Let me tell you fifty minutes of ab exercises can be a doozy! I am also working on being able to kneel on the floor and crawl around and play with Will. I have spent a lot of time practicing the crawling and kneeling and pretend picking up toys! My knees are getting a workout!

The current plan is to head back to work part-time after Memorial Day. Due to my decrease in stamina, we will ease back into working full time. I will continue outpatient therapy the days I am not at work. My boss and co-workers have been so supportive and amazing. I miss them all and look forward to getting back to see them!

I wanted to put a huge thank you out to many of you! We have been so appreciative of the meals people have brought and sent. It has made things so much easier! My mom has also been a huge help with the laundry, taking Will to school, and getting up with him every morning. Mr. Will is working on reading the numbers on the clock. "Mimi says it has to start with a six or we don't get up!"

I have spent some time the last few weeks going back through all the cards, emails, etc. that all of you sent through this ordeal. All the love and support we have received has meant so much to me. It has been quite the journey I'd say, but I have learned a lot through it all. Family is of number one importance to me and this has been a good reminder of that. With that theme in mind, have a great Mother's day and enjoy the sunshine!

Love,
Carrie

Mother's Day was another milestone to celebrate! I was not sure how much of a mother I was going to be able to be to Will after I got through GBS. I'll never forget on Christmas morning when my brother was kind enough to video chat with us while Jeff held my phone up so I could see Will open his presents from Santa. As Will smiled and giggled, my heart just sank. I wondered if I would ever be back in my house with Will for future Christmases. Those were the scary moments, the tough moments that I am so happy to be on the other side of now.

It was also very special that my mom was staying with us and could join us at the childcare Mother's Day breakfast. It sounds fancy, but actually it's muffins, fruit, and juice you enjoy while sitting on the floor with the kids. I do love the great pictures of Mimi, Will, and me that day. Will looks so proud to have us there and so happy. His smile makes me smile just thinking about it.

It was a blessing that my mom could come and stay with us for almost two months while I was in outpatient rehab. It really helped to have another set of hands in the morning to get me off to rehab and Will off to school, and then help with laundry, cooking, and the dozens of other things it takes to run a household and care for family. There are probably few married couples who can say they had a mother-in-law stay with them for two months and survived it. Kathy, you can come stay anytime! (Although we learned she's not a fan of Indian food.)

Outpatient rehab was no joke. I was just drained when it was done. They literally helped me get back on my feet. It's difficult to describe how your feet feel when you can't feel them at all when you walk. I've compared it to wearing ski boots all the time. I HATE ski boots. Frankly, I don't ski anymore because I really dislike ski boots. It's a weird feeling. So when the PT said, "Let's try running!" I thought he was crazy. Just like at RIC, the outpatient therapists knew how to get you moving, how to push you to do the one thing you dreaded or were scared to do. We also went on community excursions to help prepare us to be back out in the real world. I went shopping one day and mini golfing with a group of patients another day. These excursions really helped give me confidence that I could do everyday life again.

I hated crawling around on mats picking up toys and blankets and books, then having to stand up and walk them to a basket and do it again. But now when I am picking up toys or something else, I think back to that occupational therapy and am thankful they helped re-train my body.

July 26, 2014

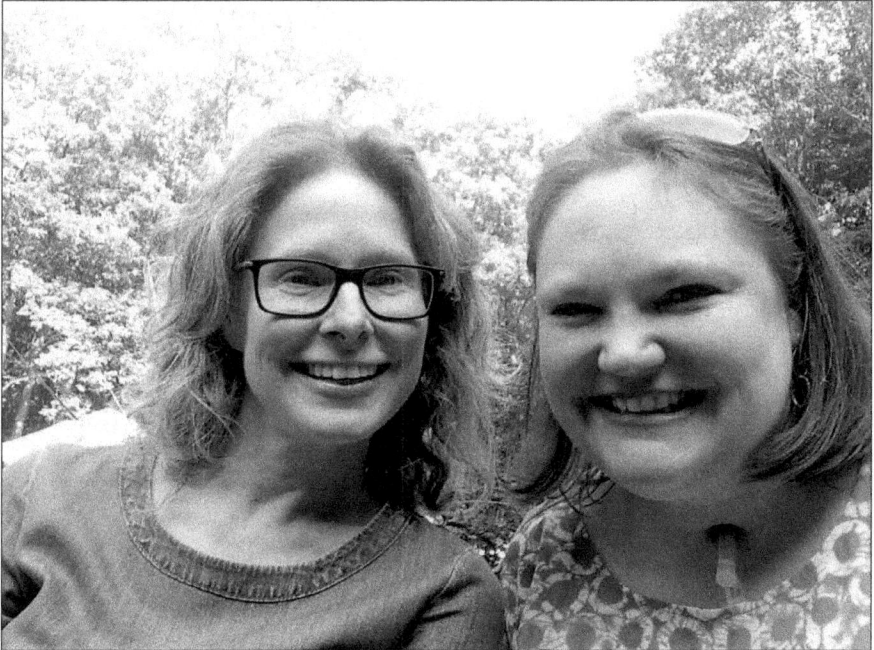

Carrie and her good friend Heather Bush at Carrie's half-birthday party! You can see the T-tube in Carrie's throat.

July 26, 2014 – Final Update from Carrie!

Howdy Friends and Family!

It has been more than two months since my last update, so I thought it would be fun to send out one last report!

I am doing great and still getting stronger day by day. We have had a super fun summer thus far with Cubs games, trips to the Libertyville pool, and throwing a little guy two fantastic Curious George birthday parties for the big number four. I am now back at work full time and have enjoyed getting back in the swing of things. My co-workers have been fantastic, not only bringing me up to speed on what I missed, but taking care of me and making sure I am not over doing it.

I graduated from therapy in late June. I'd passed all my goals and we discussed whether continuing outpatient PT was necessary.

"If you chase around your son when you get home from work then I don't think you need to continue," my PT told me.

So a few days a week, Jeff, Will, and I head over to Independence Grove, a forest preserve near our house, and walk together. I also have a few at home arm, core and ankle workouts I fit in when I can. I have been playing soccer with Will in the yard and working on my tee-ball swing! Slowly and surely, I feel like I am getting back to normal. I still have numbness in my feet and tend to get pain at night, especially if I have been on my feet a lot during the day. But the good news is I think the numbness is getting better!

A big win in our house this past week was me being able to get out of the shower by myself. As you all know, Jeff is amazing! For the last four months since I have been home, I would sit on the bench in our shower and get all cleaned up. When I finished, Jeff would come in, turn off the water, hang up the handheld showerhead, then get a towel for me to step onto. When you cannot feel your feet, it turns out getting out of a wet shower can be quite scary. This past week I felt safe enough to give it a go on my own. Success! Saves some extra laundry and gives me more freedom to shower whenever I want. Yeah me!

I want to personally thank Kent Seacrest in this email. For those of you who do not know Kent, he battled GBS about six months before I came down with it. Kent has been my mentor through this journey. He and his wife Ann came to visit me in January when I was struggling quite a bit and have stayed in touch throughout my GBS experience. I remember in January Kent saying, "I don't regret having GBS." At the time, I thought the guy was crazy. I was miserable and frustrated, but now that I have battled through it, I understand what Kent meant. I am proud to say I beat GBS, I learned a lot and understand that this was part of my life plan to go through this experience. I have been reading this book called the *Happiness Advantage* and one chapter of the book it talks about people that go through life-altering health events. Instead of just "bouncing back" from these health issues, the book discusses "bouncing forward" as the process you go through actually enriches your life. I don't ever want to go through it again, BUT am thankful to have survived GBS.

Next weekend my good friends Heather and David Bush are throwing me a half birthday party since I spent my previous birthday in the ICU! I am looking forward to celebrating with a lot of good friends and thanking them for their support. Labor Day weekend we are going back to Nebraska to visit so I look forward to seeing many of your smiling faces then.

We see the neurologist this coming Friday. On Sept. 25th I am scheduled to get the T-tube out of my throat! I look forward to putting this journey in the rearview mirror. I tell folks I am about eighty-five percent and feel like I continue to "bounce forward!" I am working on a book to highlight this journey so someday Will can sit down and read through it. Not sure if I will officially publish it, but this email clan will get the first view of the book when I finish it (guessing by 2015 sometime).

Thanks again for all your love and support.

Signing off!
Carrie

The half birthday party was amazing! Thank you to Heather and David for always throwing such fabulous parties! Dawn, a friend from work, made an amazing Wonder Woman cake and lots of other goodies that I think we enjoyed for weeks! It was so wonderful to be able to drink, eat, and enjoy the company of so many great friends who played such a key role in my recovery.

Going back to work was exciting to me. I was ready to put my mind back to use after being so focused on my body for the past six months. I work for a pharmaceutical company in an operational business group. We help our scientists and regulatory strategists focus on bringing our important therapies to the market while my team supports them in their day-to-day business needs with project management, budgeting, facilities, etc. I was nervous that I had missed so much I would not be able to jump back in. My co-workers were rock stars. Not only did they keep all the balls in the air while I was gone, so many of them went above and beyond covering my work and pushing our mission forward.

The day I went back to the office, they had a cake and a huge sign waiting for me. I was able to go back part time, taking it slow, working half days just a few days a week while I was still in therapy. It is fascinating that work goes on without you. I learned through this ordeal that everyone is replaceable, and it is a good thing. I am happy my team and co-workers could keep everything going while I was gone. I know it was hard not having my notes, my files, my help, but they did it and I owe quite a few of them a lot of drinks. My manager and friend, Heather, really helped me not worry about work. She'd assure me they were all fine. Bruno, whom I had hired just a few months before I got ill, took over our team and did a phenomenal job. I'm grateful for Lauren, Lizelle, JP, Jen, Tina, Ben, David, and so many others who carried extra workload covering for me while I was out.

When I returned to work, many of the issues seemed trivial to me after what I had endured the past six months. That is hard to explain to people who had not been with me daily on my journey. When work disagreements or issues arose, I tried to really take Kent Seacrest's words of wisdom to heart asking myself, "Will it matter in three months? If not, let it go!"

I felt like I was getting back into a groove at work, at home and in life. I was still not completely steady on my feet with the numbness, so I did end up going back to PT at a center closer to home once a week to work on balance and strength. My PT was another fiery red head who helped me get back to where I am today (about ninety-five percent). Jeff would often take Will next door to his swim lesson and then they would come over to check on me. My physical therapist was great with Will and would play games with him while I finished my exercises. I just don't think my balance or the overall feeling in my feet will ever get to 100 percent and that is okay with me. I am happy to be walking and doing normal day-to-day activities. At PT, we worked a lot on my balance. I stood on those foam things again and threw balls at a net that bounced the ball back to me. I walked toe-to-toe and stood on one leg. Since I could not feel my feet, I had to retrain my body to compensate. Eventually, I had to do box jumps, and man was I scared, but I did it! I was coming back. Today I have a few limitations. I still get really achy feet if I am really tired and, on most days, cannot fully feel my feet. I have come to accept these limitations and be aware of them in all I do.

You now understand why I named my book *Bouncing Forward*. I truly believe I have bounced forward from this experience. I learned more than I can explain in this book about myself, my strength, my fears, my abilities. And I realized how those relationships that we spend a life to build come back to you full circle when you need them most. I am confident I can handle anything life throws at me.

But my GBS journey was not completely over. We had more hurdles to face.

October 3, 2014

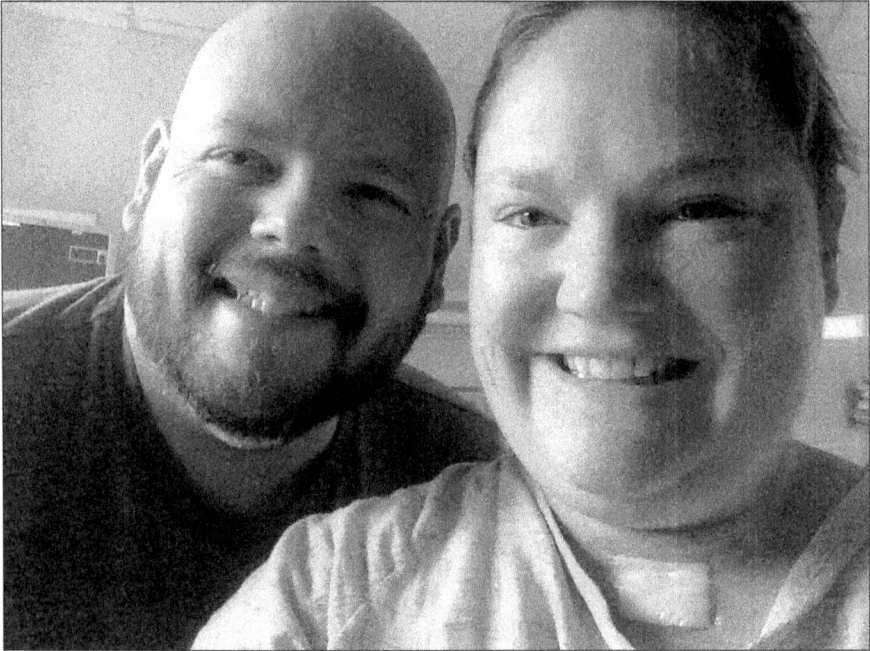

Carrie and Jeff after her T-Tube was removed smiling as they thought the trachea issues were behind them.

Fri, Oct 3, 2014 at 7:52 p.m., from Jeff's email:

Friends and Family,

I'm (unfortunately) back to sending some updates on Carrie. Last week we triumphantly went into Northwestern for what we had hoped would be the final surgery, the removal of the T-tube. Over the last week, Carrie felt like her breathing was getting more and more labored, so we went in for a follow-up with the ENT doctor. He took a look and did not like what he saw, so he immediately admitted Carrie to the ICU. The bronchoscopy showed a severe narrowing or stenosis of the windpipe, very likely due to the initial trauma from the trach, the reason we had the T-tube in the first place.

Earlier today, a non-T stent was placed in Carrie's windpipe to hold that stenosis open and allow her to breathe more easily. It went fairly well, but both surgeons mentioned that it was really tough material to work through to get the stent into place. Carrie is being held overnight and will probably be discharged tomorrow (Saturday).

The next step is for us to meet with the "big boss" who is a thoracic surgeon, who will look at all of the video and measurements from today's surgery and determine the long-term plan. Either we will have the stent in for a longer period of time (six or more months again), or we will have what is called a re-sectioning of the trachea, where a ring of "'bad" windpipe is surgically removed.

She is resting comfortably tonight, but is obviously frustrated that we don't know exactly what is happening, and how we are going to move forward to get off this hospital roller coaster.

My folks have driven up to help take care of Will until we have a better idea of the plan, but as always, we appreciate prayers and positive thoughts.

You can reach directly out to Carrie via text, email, or phone. I just wanted to let everyone know while she's recovering from a couple hours of anesthesia and the headache that inevitably follows.

Jeff

I am sitting in the ICU after having my T-tube removed. They had me stay overnight as precaution. Good news is I am still breathing! The surgery went well. I had some granulation tissue still there but with the tubes out they don't think it will grow back. Sitting up in a chair in the ICU is an odd feeling. Back in December when this was my home for three weeks, I couldn't move. Jeff spent a lot of nights sleeping on this not-comfortable-what-so-ever chair. I look around. The computer the nurse uses, the TV, the view out the window all look familiar. I have to think hard to remember how uncomfortable I was, how I could not move a muscle. I am thankful some of those memories are fading. I am just so grateful to have recovered so much in a relatively short timeframe compared to what I could have endured. Don't let me undersell it—it was still hell most of the time, but I beat the odds relatively speaking and I could not be happier about that. I was very sick, unsure if I would ever walk again, let alone drink water! Life is good.

And in the corner of my room, the cell phone is buzzing with new emails and texts. I read through them and there is an issue going on at work that is stressful. I start to feel my heart rate go up and confirm that is the case by looking at the monitors behind me. How quickly we get sucked back in to the day-to-day grind of work, responsibilities. My goal is to keep trying to maintain perspective and bring that perspective to all I do. It is very hard, but I do see change in my life.

It felt great to have that T-tube removed. I thought we were done with surgeries and hospitals and I was moving on with my life. I went back to work that next week. I remember walking into work a few days later and feeling very winded. I had to stop halfway and catch my breath. It was very odd. My head told me something was wrong; my heart didn't want to hear it. My co-workers asked if I was okay. I could see the worry on their faces. The next day was no different, so I finally called the ENT office and they told me to come in the very next day. The story was not yet over.

The ENT let me watch as he scoped my throat. "Whoa that's not good," I remember him saying. That did not look normal. My throat was reduced to a very, very small opening the size of an eraser on the end of a pencil. My ENT doctor said the opening should be the size of a half dollar. They took me into surgery that day to put a stent in to ensure I was able to breathe. I could not believe we were on surgery number seven for my delicate windpipe. I was scared that this was going to become my new normal.

October 8, 2014

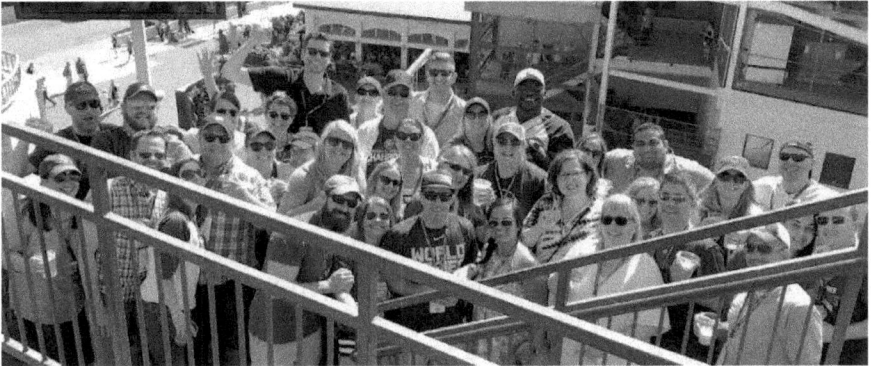

Carrie and her friends celebrating her 40ᵗʰ birthday! So many of these friends aided Carrie in her recovery.

Wednesday, October 8, 2014, from Carrie's email:

Hi Friends,

Good news: I am back to breathing normally and chasing Will around the bases in our front yard baseball games!

I got released on Saturday after they confirmed the stent was doing its job. We saw the thoracic surgeon yesterday (Tuesday) to discuss next steps. After waiting two hours to talk to him, we were thoroughly impressed and agreed to his recommended plan of attack.

On Friday, Nov.7th I will have outpatient surgery to have the stent removed. I will relax over the weekend at home and go

225

back to the hospital on Monday, Nov.10th. The thoracic surgeon will perform what is called a tracheal re-sectioning where they basically cut out the bad part of my trachea (where the narrowing or stenosis is located), then re-stitch my windpipe back together. The fun part of the surgery is that because the stenosis is lower on my windpipe, they have to do a sternotomy (cut through my sternum with a saw) to get to the windpipe which obviously adds to my recovery time. I will most likely be in the hospital for the remainder of that week (through approximately Nov.14th), then come home to recover for a few weeks.

We are happy that we have a plan of attack and that this procedure should be the best long-term fix for my trachea issues. Turns out being on a ventilator with a trachea tube in for a few months is not a good thing for your body and is what has led to these re-occurring scar tissue issues. This surgery should help solve the issues once and for all.

We appreciate all your prayers and support as we jump this (hopefully) last hurdle. My parents will be coming out for the surgery and then Jeff's mom will come to help when I get home. We will definitely let you all know how the surgeries go in November and appreciate your positive vibes!

It's not the October and November we had planned, but as Jeff says, if we can get through this fall, we can plan lots of fun trips for the next thirty years of falls!

Off to read books to Will before bed! Thanks for your love and support.

Carrie

October 29, 2014

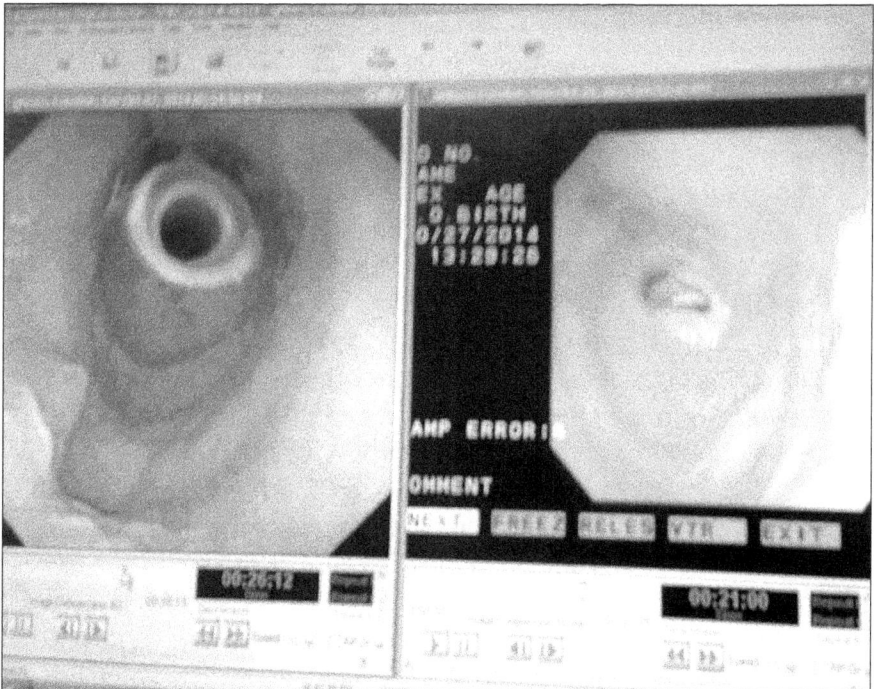

The picture on the left is Carrie's windpipe after the stent was put in. The picture on the right shows the granulation tissue and severe narrowing of Carrie's windpipe a few weeks later.

Wednesday, October 29, 2014, from Carrie's email:

Friends -

We wanted to reach out and ask for all of you to send those positive vibes and prayers. Unfortunately, our best laid plans hit another hurdle these past few days. Last Thursday, I started feeling short of breath again. My co-workers noticed that while I was trying to spout my wisdom in meetings, I would have to pause to take a big breathes every few words. (I am sure it was a good attention getter!)

I went to my ENT on Monday to get my windpipe scoped to see how it looked, and unfortunately more granulation tissue had grown above the stent they put in on Oct. 4th. So, as you might imagine, they have kept me in the hospital as I have only a pretty small area to breathe through. This is causing my shortness of breath when walking etc.

So surgery is occurring today, and we have two potential options. They will decide in the operating room as they really need to get inside my throat and assess. My ENT, the pulmonologist (who put the original stent in), and the Thoracic surgeon will all be involved in the decision on which option to pursue.

Option 1: Open up windpipe (dilate etc.) and then remove the current stent to prepare me for the re-sectioning surgery to be moved up to later this week or early next week.

Option 2: Open up the windpipe (dilate etc.) and then put a longer internal stent in to cover both stenosis (narrowing of windpipe) areas. I would then have to schedule two more surgeries: one to remove the new stent, and another to perform the re-sectioning surgery.

It all depends on how angry (flared up) my windpipe looks and what they believe is the safest course of action for me.

Dick and Kathy (my parents) arrived last night, which is super helpful. Unfortunately, we will miss a trip we had planned to Nebraska to watch Purdue try to score a touchdown against Nebraska, but there will be another trip in two years! Will was at home sick with a fever earlier this week and Jeff had strained his back two weeks ago, so our house was a little under the weather. We are hoping we are all on the road to recovery now!

Jeff or I will try to send an update tonight to let you know how things went. We are remaining positive that we are still on a path to fix this delicate flower of a windpipe. My body just must have missed the hospital so much it wanted to have a few extra stays.

Thanks for your friendship and support. I cannot express how critical my support network has been in my recovery. I feel so lucky!

Love,

Carrie and Jeff

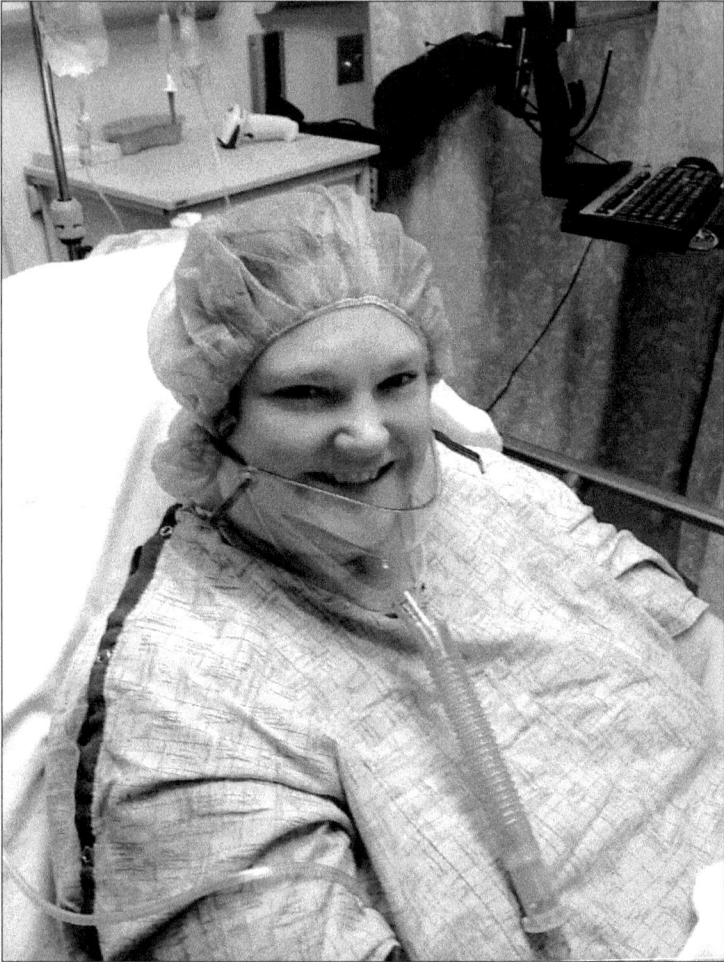

Carrie ready for Surgery!

Wednesday, October 29, 2014, from Carrie's email:
Surgery Update from today

Friends -

Thank you for all the kind notes, words of wisdom, and happy thoughts!

They all paid off!

I am resting comfortably in my room and am scheduled to have the windpipe re-sectioning surgery on Friday around noon. All three doctors (I am good hands!) met with Jeff post-surgery and said they were happy to find the stent had actually moved down in my windpipe so the narrowing of the airway they saw Monday was actually the original problem area. This turns out to be really good news because right before they took me into surgery today, they said that if it was new stenosis (narrowing) then I would most likely not be a candidate for the re-sectioning and they were probably going to put a T-tube back in for at least a year. That was pretty tough news to hear right before surgery, but I thought of all the positive vibes sent my way, and we got the best outcome. They realized the stent had slipped, so they removed it, dilated the problem area to buy me a few days to let my windpipe calm down, and agreed to move forward with the re-sectioning!

The next surgery on Friday is more serious. They will cut out the bad part and then stretch my windpipe as much as they can. They found out today that the length of the bad area in my windpipe is longer than they had hoped, so again, they will not know the full plan until they get into the operating room and see my windpipe to determine the "tricks up their sleeves" they will use. I feel very confident in the thoracic surgeon and am hopeful this will come out positively! They will still need to saw through my sternum to get to the windpipe so I will be in hospital through next week sometime with a fun stitch from my chin to my chest to keep that windpipe from pulling.

I am not sure when I'll feel like having visitors, so feel free to reach out to me and I will let you know if I am getting bored and need friends or if you better stay away because I am having a tough day!

I love your notes and your stories, as we have all struggled through our own journeys and have words of wisdom to share.

Jeff will most likely send the next update Friday night or Saturday.

Off to rest as the doctor says!
Carrie

PS: Big thanks to my parents who are going to stay through next week to help us through the surgery and hospital time. Mr. Will is going to be Spiderman tomorrow night and go trick or treating with Papa. Jeff and I are bummed to be Skyping another holiday with our son ☺, but we are hopeful it will be the last one! 2015 is going to be our year!

October 31, 2014

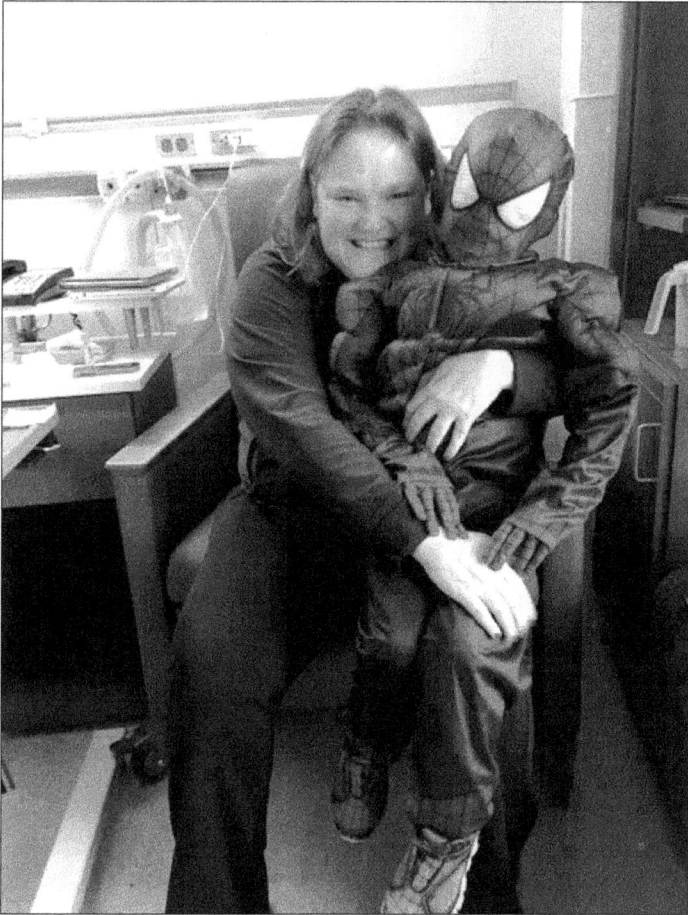

Will (as Spider-Man) visiting Carrie in the hospital before her surgery.

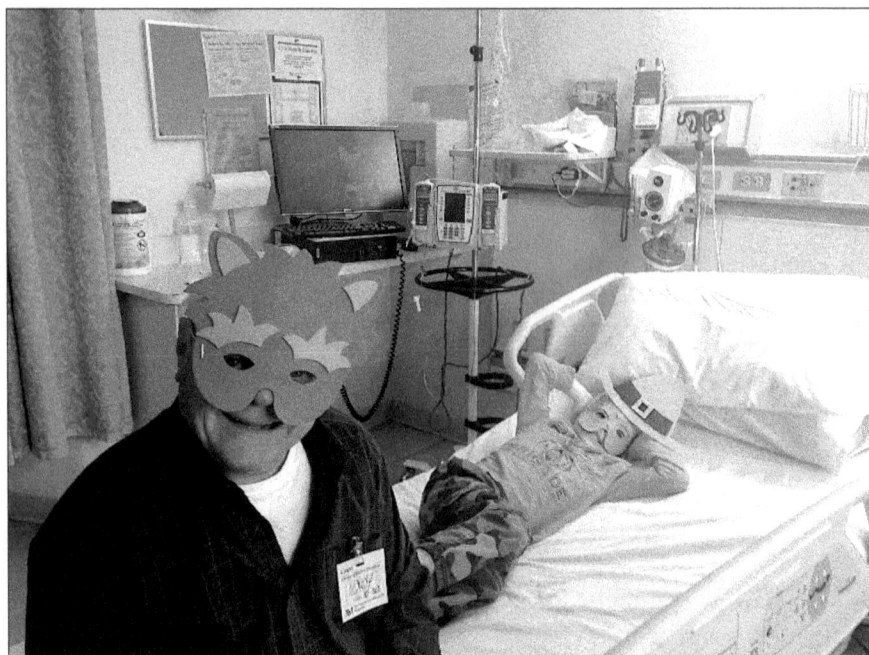

*Dick (Carrie's Dad) and Will wearing Halloween masks
in Carrie's hospital room.*

Friday, October 31, 2014, from Jeff's email:

Carrie wanted me to get a quick note out to everyone this evening.

She went into surgery at roughly 1:00 p.m. and was finished shortly before 5:00. The thoracic surgeon told me he only resected approximately two centimeters of trachea and that everything went well. He only needed to perform a partial or median sternotomy, which should help with her recovery time. The reconnection of the trachea went very smoothly, and did not require any of the "tricks" we had discussed, so that was a great relief to Carrie—no concerns about not being able to eat or having to go back to speech/swallow therapy.

She is resting, not particularly comfortably, in the ICU at Northwestern, just a door away from where we spent a long two weeks last December. The hope is that by tomorrow we'll get her back on her feet and into a regular non-ICU room. Her vitals are great and she's hitting the pain med button every fifteen minutes, so I know she's hurting.

Her breathing is strong and there are no indications of undue bleeding, other than the disaster of an arterial IV that they put in during the surgery, but that should come out in the next couple of days and is purely for on-demand blood pressure monitoring.

She wanted to tell everyone that we appreciate the many, many emails and calls and texts. We're trying to respond to all of them.

Mr. Will braved the chilly winds and managed to trick or treat the length of our block at home with Papa, and is currently enjoying his spoils and some McNuggets. We both sincerely hope this is the very last holiday interrupted by surgery.

Jeff

November 6, 2014

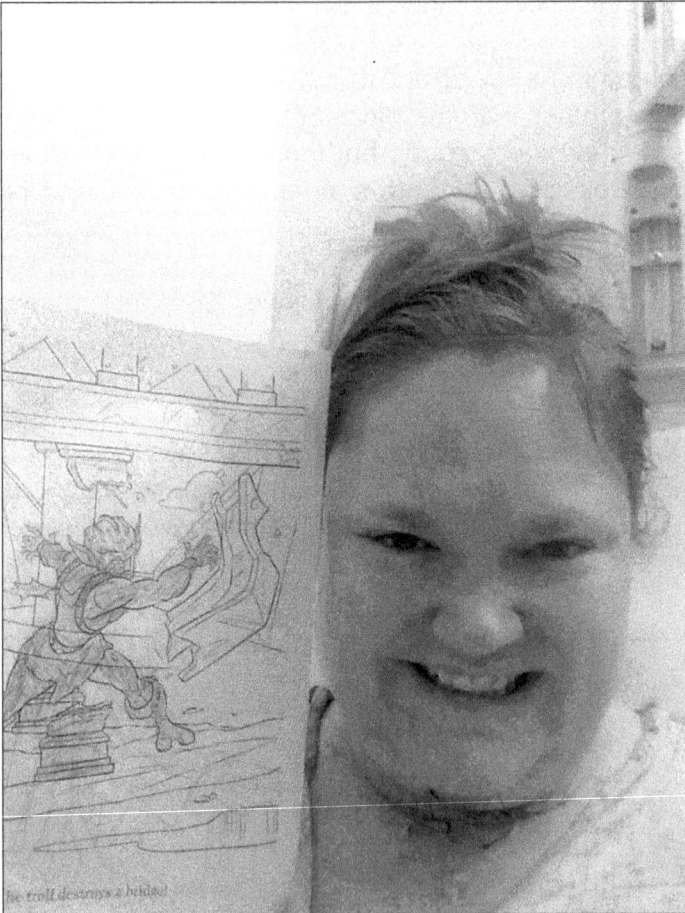

Carrie after tracheal resection holding picture Will colored for her.
See stitch from her chin to chest.

Nov 6, 2014, at 1:07 p.m., from Carrie's email:

Hi Friends -

Our hope was to be sending a note out last night that I had been released from the hospital and all was great. Unfortunately, there were a few more setbacks to overcome on this windpipe journey—all manageable though so that is the good news!

First of all, they did a scoping of my windpipe yesterday to make sure everything was healing well and there was not any additional narrowing of the airway, etc. Great news! The scope was very clear and everything is healing nicely!

The original plan was for me to go home yesterday (Nov. 5th). Earlier in the week, I started having the chills and popped a 103.1 temperature. After some tests, we learned I had unfortunately sprung an infection in my neck wound. A CAT scan confirmed that the infection is centralized to that area, so we are managing the problem location. The goal is to ensure I am fever free for twenty-four hours and have a plan to take care of the wound when I go home.

Dr. Jeff enters the scene from stage right! Have I mentioned how amazing my husband is and how he has taken such good care of me? This morning they asked me if I had someone at home who could care for my wound. My response was "I have a four-year-old who would love to have that job, but I think we will have to utilize my husband's skills for my safety!" So the goal now is for them to let me go home either Friday or Saturday. We will have a home nurse visit every day for a while to check in on Dr. Jeff's work and to make sure there are no issues.

On Monday night when I was talking to Will on the phone, he said, "Mom, I think it's about time you came home now!" It was so endearing. We were bummed to have to explain that the doctors needed to keep Mommy a few more days because she had a fever. He seemed to think that made sense.

Thanks for your continued support and care.

Carrie, Jeff and want-to-be doctor Will

November 7, 2014

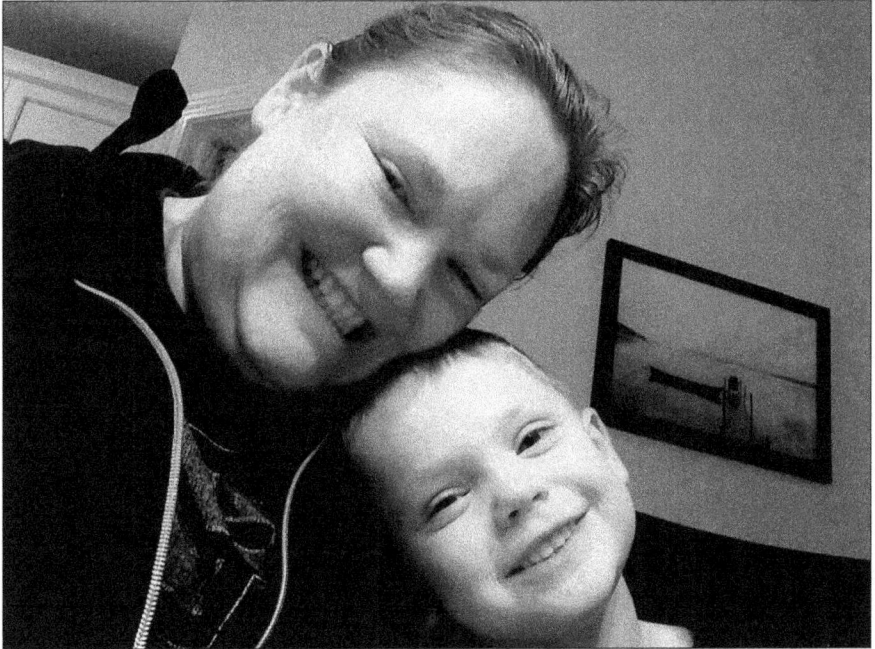

Mom is home!

Nov. 7, 2014, from Carrie's email:

We are home!

Happy Friday to all! We arrived home about 5:00 p.m. tonight. Hooray! Thanks to my parents who trekked from Libertyville all the way to downtown this week to entertain me and bring me home today! Will bought me some gorgeous orange flowers, cupcakes and a box of Spider-Man crackers (for himself, he told me!). We enjoyed a home-cooked meal and a little movie night together.

After a much-needed shower, I'm now lying in bed after multiple pillow arranging attempts by my a-number-one husband! We hope for good sleep and a relaxing weekend. The infection is being treated by antibiotics and some fun wound packing. We have our home health nurse coming tomorrow.

Jeff continues to remind me that I need to rest as I did have major surgery, but they also want me to walk multiple times a day! So, feel free to come visit and we can go for a walk around my neighborhood or I'll make you take me to Independence Grove. I cannot drive while I'm on all the pain meds!

Jeff's mom, Ardie, is coming on Monday to help out which will be great. Will just loves having more play buddies!

Love
Carrie, Jeff, and Will

I thought the emails painted a pretty good picture of the back-and-forth dance we did between home, work, and the hospital that fall. I was so excited to get my T-tube out and move on with life. I saw it as the last hurdle and realized I was not running a 100-meter hurdle event but the 400-meter hurdles. I kept having to reset my expectations, which is hard to do when you have endured what you believe is enough. The good news is I had great care with my doctors and felt very confident in their advice and what they wanted to do. In the end the trachea re-sectioning was the key to my delicate flower of a windpipe issues going away for good.

I have a pretty cool battle scar from the cracking of my sternum. I often find people looking at my scar, wanting to ask. Few people do ask about it though, which is interesting to me. I am happy to tell the story and actually appreciate the opportunity to talk about what I endured to get that battle scar. I am proud of what I went through, and proud to show off my scar. Will told me it made me a super hero and that made me extra proud. I feel like a super hero – battling GBS and smashing it to the curb!

EPILOGUE

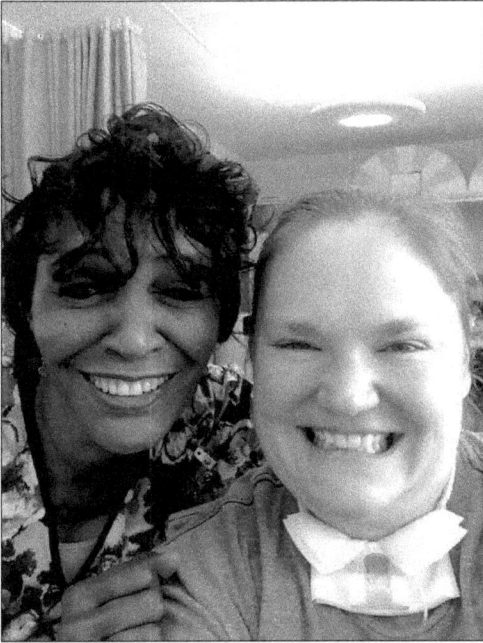

Left: Carrie with nurse Laurana.

Below: Carrie with PCT Stephanie.

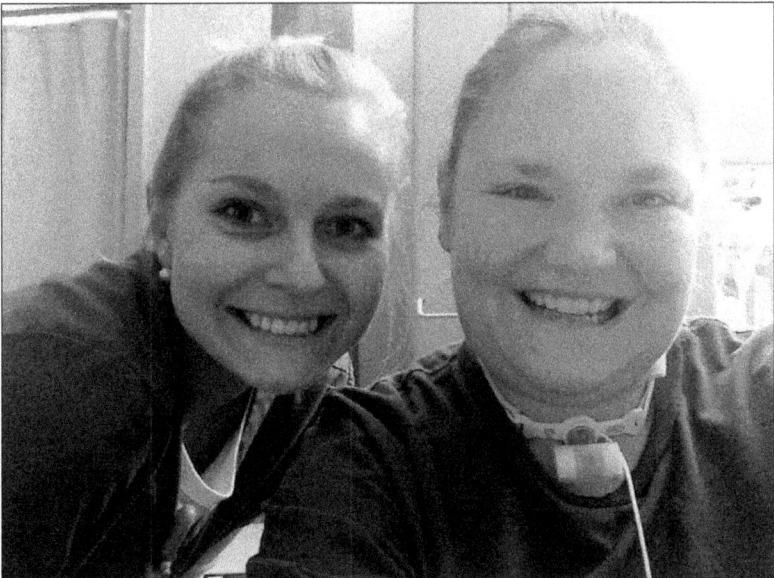

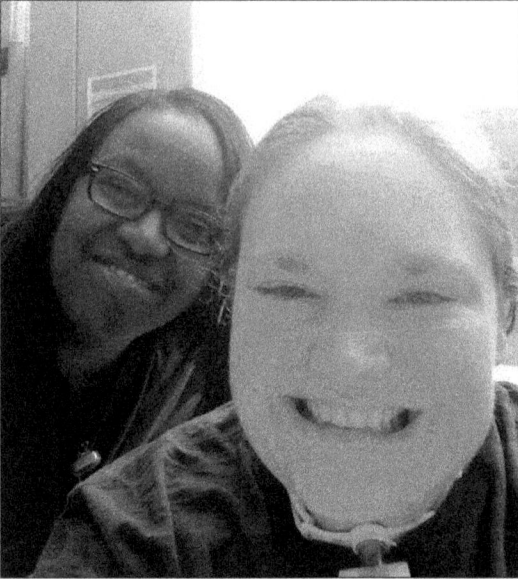

Left:
Carrie with
nurse Crystal.

Below:
Carrie with PT
Martha.

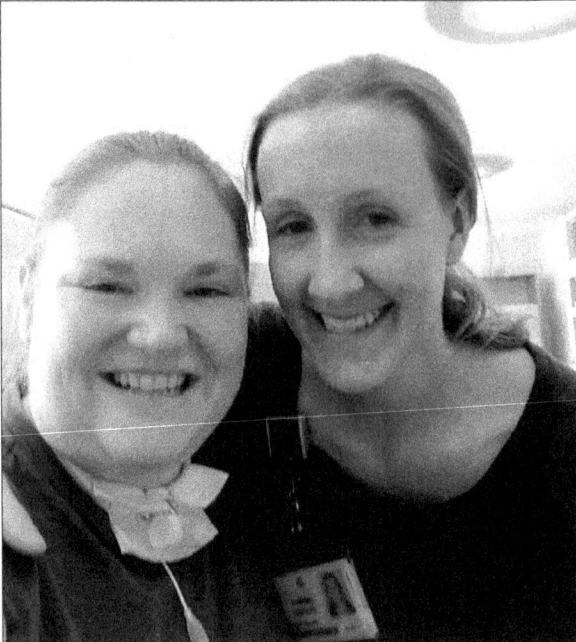

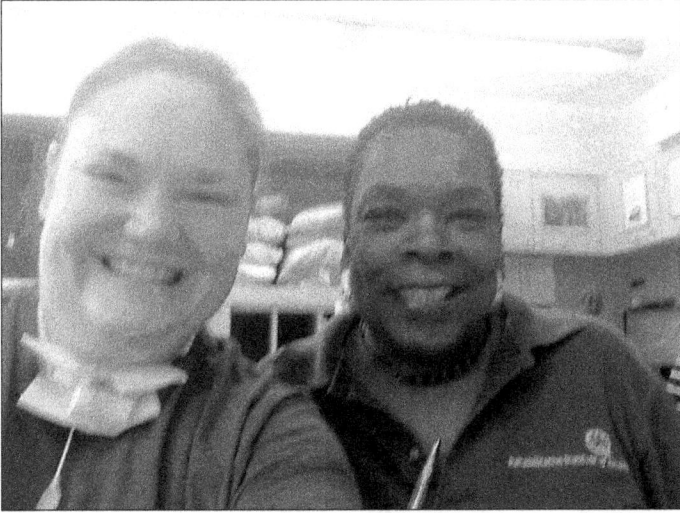

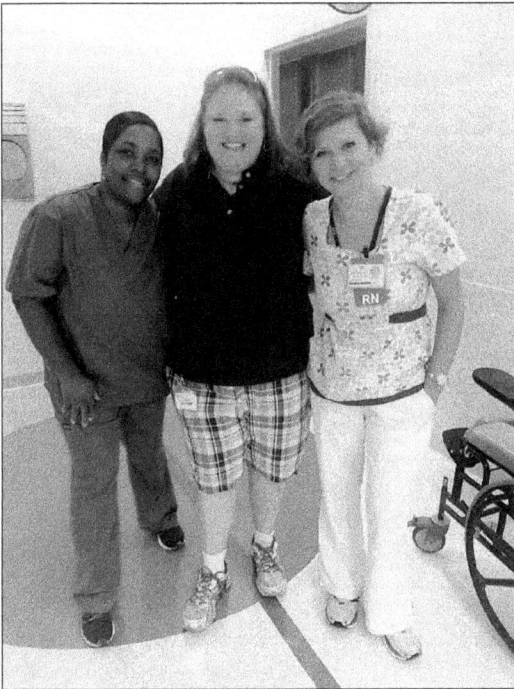

Above: Carrie with the "tooth fairy."

Left: Visiting RIC in Summer 2014 with PCT Vanessa and nurse Sonia.

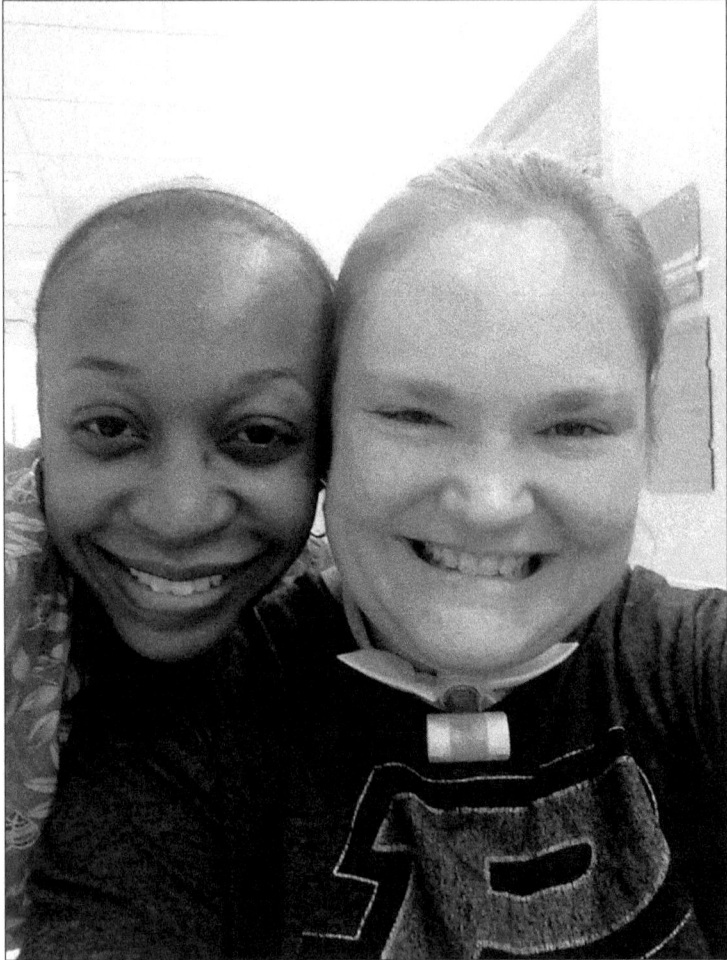

Carrie and PCT Mary.

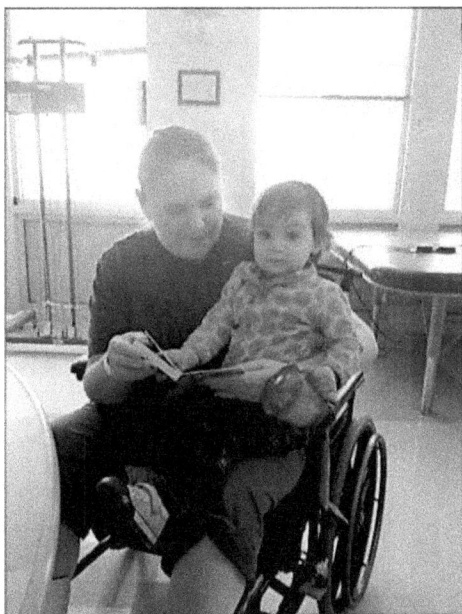

Left: Carrie reading a book to Brooklyn, Carrie's cousin Mandy's daughter.

Bottom: Some of Carrie's cousins – Mandy, Chris, Amy, Carrie, Sarah, and Suzanne who were a supportive force during her battle.

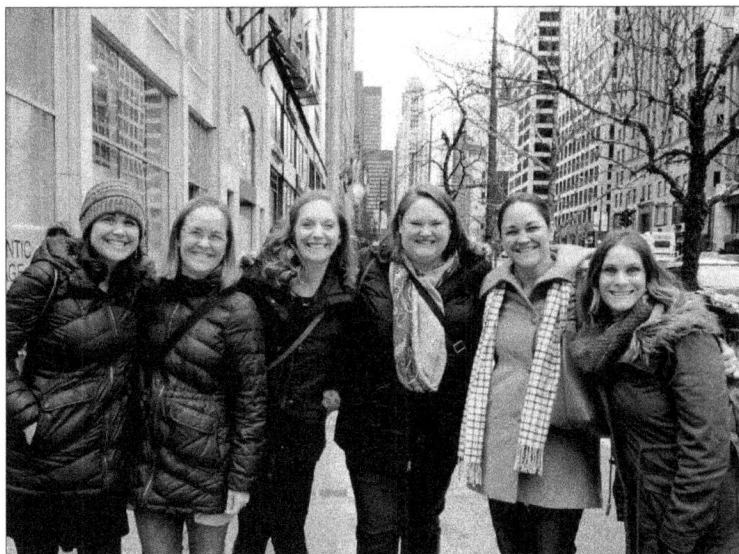

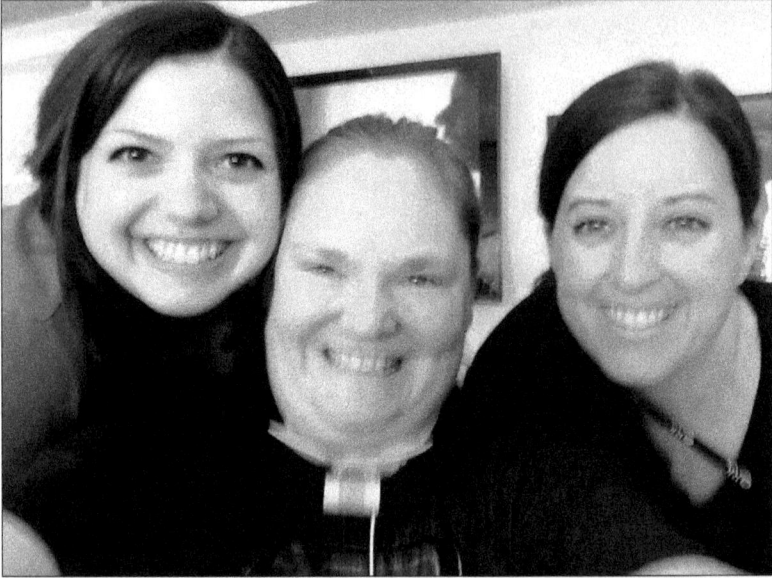

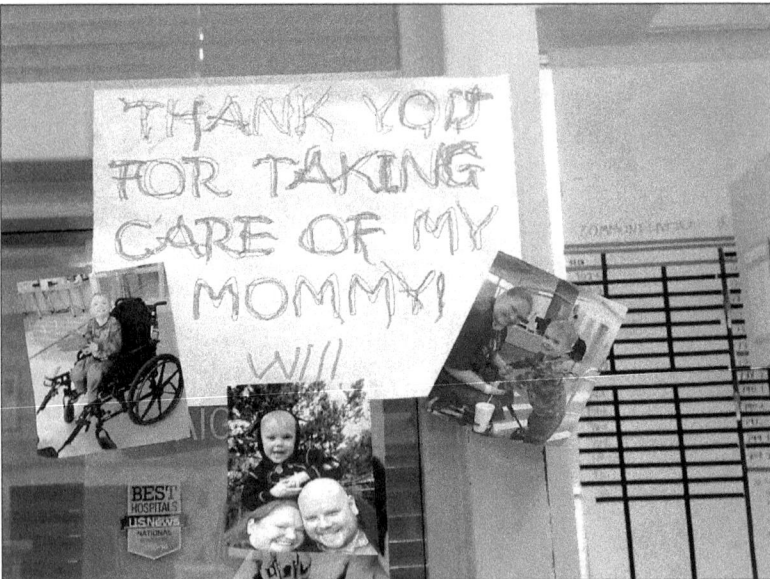

Top: Zoe, Carrie and OT Jessica.
Bottom: Sign Will (and Dad) made for the nurses and PCTs.

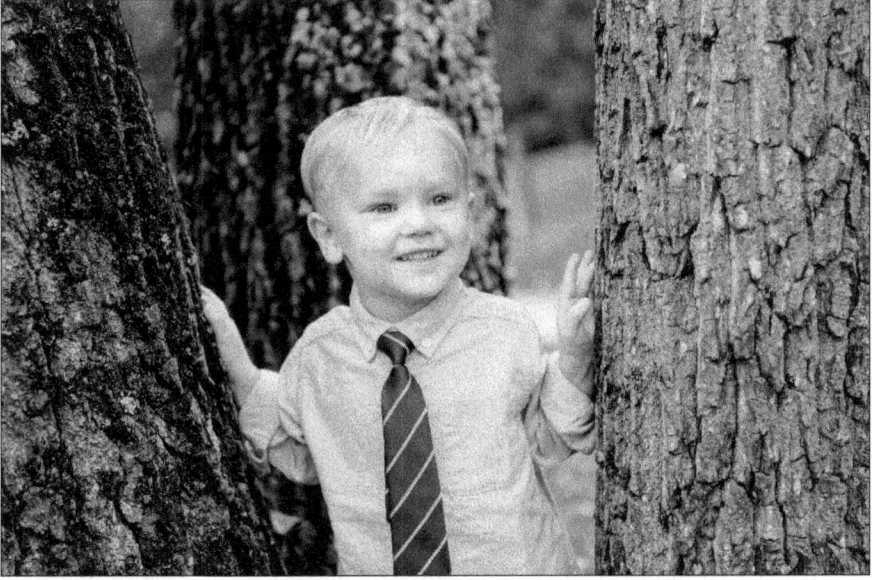

Zach – Born April 2016

So turns out I didn't quite get the book done in 2015. It's 2018 as I am editing these final chapters, but I am confident 2019 is the year! It seems living life and spending as much time with my family as possible took time away from completing the book.

Unfortunately, since I started writing this book, Jeff and I have had other ups and downs. Before I got GBS, we had been doing fertility treatments and trying to have another baby. They wanted my body to have some time to heal and regain strength before resuming those activities. We got the all clear the beginning of 2015 and went back at it. (I meant we went back to the doctor. What were you thinking?) We resumed intrauterine insemination (IUI). I have one bad side where my tubes basically went to a black hole and so if the biggest egg was on this side, it was a no go that month. That was the case for three months, and I was getting pretty frustrated. Then we had a few months when it didn't take. We were debating how long we would try. I was in Germany for work getting ready to fly home. I took a pregnancy test and bam! We were pregnant.

We went to see the fertility doctor and he did an ultrasound. He turned to us and said, "How do you feel about having twins?" We were shocked! We knew it was a possibility but had not fully contemplated it. We were just hoping we could get pregnant.

The first trimester was tough. I had some heavy bleeding about eight weeks in. I had a placenta abruption where the placenta starts to pull away from the uterine lining. They checked and the babies looked fine but asked that I refrain from coaching Will's soccer team and working out strenuously. I followed the doctors' orders, and at our fifteen-week checkup, they did another ultrasound and said both babies looked great. We were out of the danger zone. They encouraged me to still take it easy but felt like the issue had resolved.

We were devastated when we went to our eighteen-week checkup and found out one of the babies did not have a heartbeat and had passed away. I am not sure any parent is ever prepared to hear those words. Our doctor's office was at the hospital which was so helpful as a counselor came and talked to us to help us process this information. We discussed how to explain the baby passing to Will, who was so excited to be a big brother to two babies.

It was a hard time for our family. We will always think of baby B who passed. I had hoped GBS was the worst thing my family and I would have to endure, but I have come to learn that there will be many difficult situations in life we have to work through. I believe how we react to these difficulties and how we come through helps us in bouncing forward.

We are so fortunate today to have a healthy baby boy, Zachary Barton, who was born on April 21, 2016. Zachary was the second twin who survived. He is full of energy and smart as ever, always finding the one thing he is not supposed to play with. Will is a fantastic big brother, except for all the times he has already tackled his baby brother or the time he dropped Zach on his head. I am confident he is just toughening Zach up for the wrestling matches to come. I feel lucky to have such a fun loving and healthy family after all we conquered over the past few years.

I want to make sure to thank many family and friends who helped me bounce forward. It was hard not to have family living nearby, but you learn very quickly how great your network of friends and family is when you suffer a life-altering event like GBS. Our parents gave up a lot to be by our sides through this ordeal. My parents rushed out when I first got sick and Jeff said, "I need you to come." They knew if Jeff said those words, they in fact needed to come. And Jeff's parents stayed with us multiple months in the winter while Jeff would go back and forth to the hospital and my parents needed to be in Nebraska for work. We appreciate all that our families did to help me recover and support Jeff and Will. We could not have done it without them.

Our siblings, near and far, also provided great support. Andy visited a few times with my parents—always offering a good joke to lighten the mood. Jeff's sisters, Charise and Lynette, sent gifts and cards that always brought a smile to my face. Charise sent a super comfy orange blanket. Once I got over being hot, I used it every night in the hospital. The stitching on the blanket said, "Sending hugs your way." Whenever the nurses would spread it on me at night, they would always read the stitching and make sure it was facing me so I could see it. It's the little things that helped me get better day by day.

I am just in awe of my friends. I remember being so worried that I would be alone in my hospital room, unable to call for a nurse because I did not have the strength or movement to push the call button. But I did not spend a night by myself in the hospital before I was ready. Someone from my group of friends was always by my side, staying with me when Jeff would go home for a night with Will. They still joke about the clicking sound I made to get their attention, and how annoying it was. Brooke was the best massage therapist a friend could ask for. She was always willing to rub my legs and it helped a ton. Laura was pregnant while I was in RIC and she was a trooper. Nurses would come in when she was spending the night, stop what they were doing and have a fifteen-minute conversation about her pregnancy, how it was going etc. Laura would tell them it was no big deal and that they should help me! Laura also won the award for getting me in trouble with my doctor at RIC. I was not supposed to be drinking water, but I would convince my friends to wet that sponge and let me suck on it. Laura bragged to my doctor that I sucked an entire glass of water that way the night before. Those darn sponges were taken away from me that day. I was so mad at Laura! But I love how proud of me she was.

Jennifer would bring me up to speed on pop culture and current events. I'll never forget that she slept in her coat. Even though it was zero degrees outside, I asked them to keep my room as cold as possible because I was so hot. Even though Patty was further away, she came to visit me a few times, at first always on the eighteenth of the month. During one of her visits, a few others joined us, and they had some wine that night and toasted to my recovery. I was not allowed to have any (still couldn't even drink water at the time), but I thought it was super fun!

Numerous other family members and friends were beyond helpful. The Bushes watched Will when we had to run to the emergency room early on, and helped me settle back into the house. Heather made tons of food for my family while I was in the hospital and when I returned. Meg brought food and books for my family to read, and made origami flowers for my ICU room, since real flowers weren't allowed, and then for my room at RIC. People were always so impressed by the crafty person who made those flowers.

My cousin Mandy was the best company one could have in a hospital room—just sitting and showing her support. I swear it was the quietest we Campbells have ever been. (Just ask Jeff!) Then there was my good friend Shipley who kept the Baptist women from staying another hour at my bedside when I felt horrible And Lunzmann, who flew from Nebraska for my birthday. It was the worst birthday of my life, but it was so wonderful to see her. I am just glad she got to go out with my friends that night for a cocktail and have a little fun! Bridget traveled from Nashville for the weekend and flew into my hospital room with her biggie Diet Coke and began asking questions to be sure that I was getting the best care possible! Dan Spencer, my second brother, came all the way from Denver to spend the weekend with me and Will. We laughed a lot that weekend about my crazy roommate who always wanted to chat Dan up. (I think she thought he was cute!) And who can forget the three-foot toy puppy Dan stuffed in an extra suitcase and hauled to Chicago for Will? Only marvelous friends do things like that! The visit from the Seacrests from Nebraska was a critical turning point in my recovery. I'm so thankful we had their friendship to help guide us through GBS.

Numerous other visitors came to spend time with me and fill me in on the news outside the hospital. I think Lauren and Lizelle win awards for most frequent visitors from work. They were always bringing new cards and the gossip from the office to cheer me up. There was a crew on my birthday including Meg, Tina, Heather and Lizelle who had funny hats and mustaches. (I was not looking my best, so I am glad they came back again.) Jen also came to visit, one time with Meg, Heather and David. Another time I remember Lauren bringing Jackie Montgomery who had traveled from the UK for work and was so kind to visit. The Hutchinsons, Gail and Alan Anderson, Bruno, the Trieloffs, Megan, Hrishi and Sam, Teder, Boule... I am sure there are countless others I am forgetting to mention who all came to see me, and for that I am dearly sorry. All of these incredible people took time to visit me either in the ICU or the rehab hospital. I am sure they got more than they bargained for, seeing me in a tough state, or getting coaxed into massaging my legs or trying to read my lips. But the sign of a true friend (which these folks all are) is that they just smiled and did their best to make me feel comfortable, and reassured me I would get through this. Thank you, thank, you, thank you all!

I also had phenomenal care from my nurses, PCTs, therapists, and doctors. When I first arrived at RIC, a seasoned nurse who was quiet and a little scary, Laurana, went to bat for me and found a larger bed on another floor which made turning me and getting me in and out so much easier. She became one of my favorites and I am still friends with her and so many others on Facebook. Another nurse, Sonia, worked so, so hard to make me feel human again. She would brush my hair and make it into pigtails or Princess Leia buns. People always knew when Sonia was my nurse! Kristin was so down to Earth and could always relate since she had been a patient before. Julia had a little boy the same age as Will and I loved talking to her. She was the kind of gal I knew I would be friends with outside of work. There are numerous other nurses I want to thank: James, Mary, Andrea, Crystal, and Lindsay. I also had great Patient Care Technician (PCT) care from so many people: Stephanie, Mary, Linda, Kerry, Kenya, Syed, and many, many more. I saw many additional physical and occupational therapists who helped accelerate my recovery—thank you Martha, Jessica, and countless others.

Do you remember when you went away to summer camp and every day you would wait with bated breath to see if your name got called when mail was delivered? Or was that just me? That is how it felt when I got mail at RIC. I would come back from rehab, tired, ready to get in bed, and I would see mail sitting there. Early on when I was still paralyzed to my shoulders, I would have to wait until Jeff or one of my friends came to visit so they could open the mail. I remember sometimes saving it until after dinner or until after they got me ready for bed, so I had something to look forward to. I loved getting mail!

I'll never forget the care package that the Pruetts sent. It had a huge sign that Jeff later hung in my room. It gave the white walls some much needed color! They also sent that jar of

Hershey's Kisses with a sign that read "Nurse bait!" and you know what – it worked! Doctors, nurses, PCTs all loved a little candy when they came in! Tina Lewis sent a card every week I was in the hospital and her cards always made my day. Another co-worker, Cassie, found the funniest (and often most inappropriate) cards and sent them to me. They always gave me a chuckle. She knew my humor. I got tons of cards from the Southern Heights Presbyterian Church family in Lincoln where Jeff and I were married, and my parents are members. It was so cool to hear from so many families from our church. My Aunt Carol and Aunt Ann sent me lots of cards and gifts to keep my spirits up.

And this doesn't include all the cards from cousins, friends, and family friends. All of these messages, gifts, cards, and visits demonstrated the support of the cheerleaders I had near and far. Feeling that love was reassuring and comforting. Bottom line: all of you were critical to my recovery.

Numerous nurses and therapists told me I got better for three reasons: my husband, my network of friends and family, and my positive attitude and belief that I was going to get better. Anne Marie, my occupational therapist, said that she worked with a lot of couples. She said she could tell the couples that were the real deal and, "You and Jeff are it. Booya!"

I want to add a fourth to their list: my care team (therapists, nurses, PCTs, doctors, patients, tooth fairy). They showed such respect for me as a person. I could tell in their hearts they wanted me to get better and would do whatever they could to help me achieve that goal.

I am writing the last of this book in the beautiful setting of St. Lucia. Jeff and I are here on our tenth wedding anniversary trip after coming here on our honeymoon. It is just as gorgeous and stunning as I remember it ten years ago. It's a good time to reflect on the last decade: our wedding, moving to Chicago (Evanston), our careers, the birth of our son Will, the GBS adventure, the trachea saga, the birth of our son Zach and the passing of our other baby. On a jazz cruise last night someone asked about my scar. He had his own scars from burns he endured from a fire. We all have scars and I am proud to tell the story of my scars. They mean I fought through to be able to tell this story of how I bounced forward from GBS!

Memories from Friends and Family

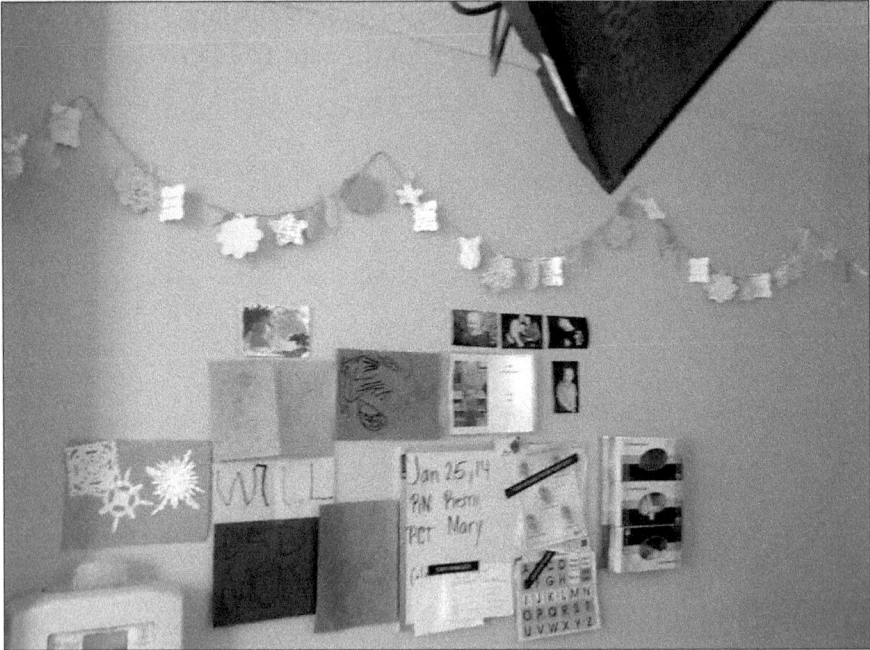

Carrie's wall at the rehab hospital with all the special notes of encouragement including the banner from the Pruetts!

I asked some of my close friends and family members to share their stories and memories from my days with GBS. It is so interesting to hear their perspectives and to learn about things I had no idea were going on during this time. So many people helped me through this journey, and this is their story too. My web of friends and relatives lived GBS step by step with me.

From Dick Campbell
Carrie's Dad

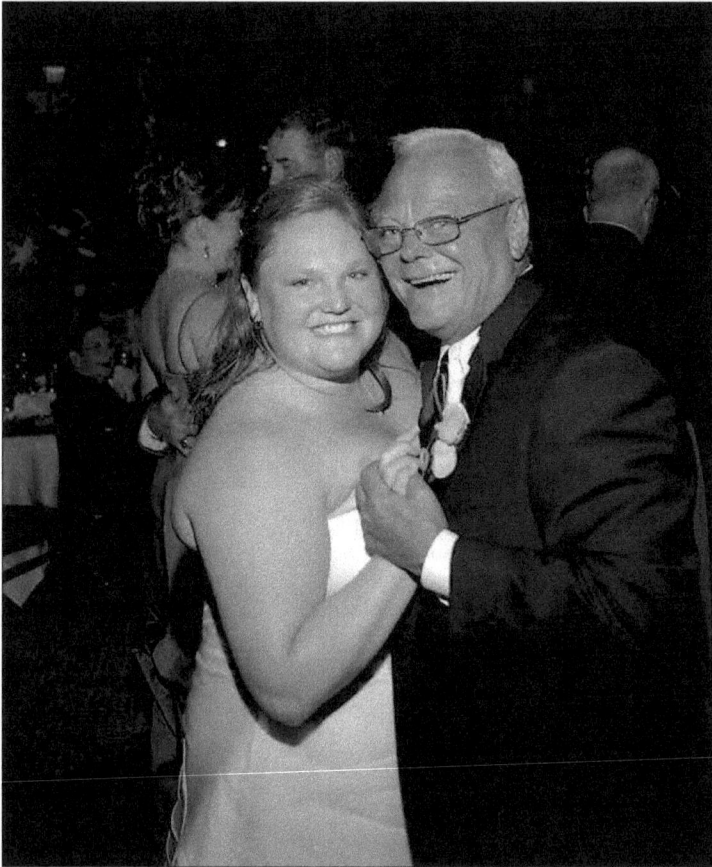

Carrie and her father, Dick, dancing at Carrie's wedding.

A Parent's Worst Fear.

On Monday December 9, 2013, at approximately 11:30 am, we received a call from our son-in-law, Jeff, that our daughter, Carrie, was in Northwestern Hospital in Lake Forest, Illinois.

By 2:00 p.m., Kathy and I were packed, in the car, and headed to Illinois. We reached Jeff and Carrie's home at ten that night. As we were driving, we were calling people to cancel appointments and meetings as we did not know when we would return home.

The next morning, we took our grandson, Will (three years old), to his childcare school and immediately headed to the hospital to see Carrie and Jeff. We walked in to find a very sick daughter. By the time we got there, the medical staff had completed a spinal tap to confirm she had Guillain-Barré, an auto-immune syndrome. The doctors had started one of the two treatments that could help her body build back immunities to fight off the nerve killing disease.

By Thursday afternoon, the treatment was not stopping the progression of the paralysis. The chief neurologist at the main downtown Chicago Northwestern Hospital wanted her transferred to that hospital as they had greater resources than the Lake Forest Hospital. Once the ambulance arrived, Kathy rode with the paramedics and I followed in the car behind them. Kathy called to suggest I not try to keep up as they were going to use lights and sirens. Also, the ambulance traveled along the shoulders of the road to get Carrie there as quickly as possible. Obviously if I followed, I would no doubt have gotten a ticket.

When I arrived, Carrie was already in the neurology ICU. Both Kathy and I were impressed with the nursing staff in the ICU. Each nurse has a maximum of two patients and work twelve-hour shifts. Thus, Carrie had the same day nurse and same night nurse except for days off. They were so attentive. The night nurse told us one evening that she felt Carrie's urine looked cloudy. She had sent it to the lab and caught a bladder infection at the earliest stage.

It is very difficult to see one of your children going through such a terrible situation, but we kept our thoughts and prayers on her improving and recovering. Little did we know how long this process would take and the strength and courage we'd see from Carrie.

Since Jeff and Carrie had planned to be Lincoln for Christmas, all of their gifts had been shipped to Nebraska. After her condition began to stabilize at the ICU, Kathy and I drove back to Lincoln to pick up our son Andy and all the presents. We returned to Chicago to stay with Will and celebrate Christmas as best we could. We Skyped with Carrie and Jeff as Will was opening his presents Christmas morning. We took a few of Carrie's presents and Will to the hospital to see his mom. As she was paralyzed, it would be three more months before she would be recovered enough to give him a hug. That tugged at us, but just in the few days we were away, we could see some recovery when we returned. Very small but celebrated victories. We stayed until Carrie was transferred to the Rehabilitation Institute of Chicago (RIC) in late December.

Over the next year, we would make nine trips to Chicago anywhere from extended weekends to Kathy staying for two and half months to assist when Carrie came home from RIC. Each trip, we saw improvement in her ability to regain the function in her limbs. First, the ability to lift an arm a little, to moving some fingers, and to eventually being able to walk around the floor with a walker. Her goal was to walk out of RIC under her own power and she did so with her walker.

As she progressed in her recovery, I would take videos with my phone. One day Carrie just shook her head, no don't do that, since she still couldn't talk. When she went back to work a couple of days a week, her manager told her that she wanted to call a team meeting and have her educate everyone as to what she had been through. Of course, that immediately brought an email: *Dad, please forward all the videos to me for my presentation!*

Outpatient rehab started with five days a week and, after several weeks, was cut back to four days a week. Finally, Carrie was able to get her trach taken out and a stent put in to keep her airway open. This was all working until the stent slipped and she was unable to breathe properly. After a few weeks of dealing with the airway problem, the doctors decided to operate on her airway, take out the weakened section and reattach the rest of the airway. To accomplish this, they had to crack open her chest, pulling ribs back to get to the airway for the repair. Fortunately, the surgery went well and there was enough airway to connect back together. Another two months of recovery!

We are so fortunate. Today, you would not know Carrie had gone through this long ordeal and has fully recovered. The full year from December 2013 to the end of 2014, was not only a struggle for Carrie and Jeff, but also for us as parents. We were constantly worried about her full recovery. We feel very blessed and know that all the prayers from family and friends and the support network that assisted Carrie during her rehab were strong contributors to the recovery of a very determined and goal-oriented woman. Her husband, Jeff, was her rock and stability. We knew she had married a great man, but he proved it over and over during that year of recovery.

And, we are blessed with a second grandson and a totally recovered daughter!

From Brooke Anderson Carrie's Best Friend

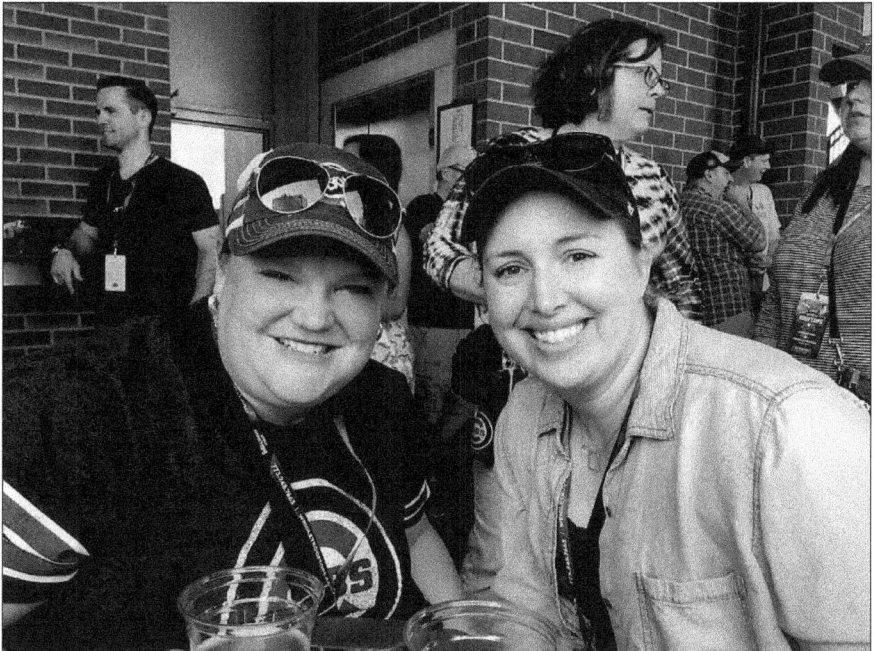

Brooke and Carrie at a Cubs game celebrating Carrie's 40th birthday!

First Things First.

There are a few things you need to know about my best friend, Carrie Campbell Grimes, in order to fully appreciate her experience and triumph over GBS. Thing One: she is an unstoppable force. I do not mean that as some trite platitude. We've been friends for more than twenty years. In college, we were pretty much inseparable. So much so that when we were going to different cities upon graduation, more than a few people questioned our ability to thrive apart. (Spoiler: we managed just fine.) So, when I tell you she is an unstoppable force, I know what I'm talking about.

Thing Two: in addition to being an unstoppable force, which is nothing to sneeze at, she exists within and exudes, this shiny, warm, nearly intoxicating sphere of energy. If I tried to describe it by color, it would be bright orange. Without a doubt. Carrie's favorite color is orange. Her affinity to orange is atypical for most adults. For starters, she has brilliant copper red hair. Beyond that, she wants *everything* in orange. Sure, the normal stuff like clothes, shoes, and the occasional bag, but she takes it to a whole other level. She's painted the walls in her bathroom orange. She currently drives an orange vehicle. And, my personal favorite, one of her wedding colors was orange. She had six bridesmaids in orange dresses! Suffice to say, Carrie's favorite color perfectly correlates to this special, special aura she has. Or maybe her favorite color is orange because she's so warm and caring and vibrant. It suits her. That is for certain.

Now, when you combine Thing One and Thing Two in one person, you get someone absolutely extraordinary. This is not a difficult or nuanced observation for someone to make about

Carrie. Rather, it pretty much hits you upside the head the moment you meet her. This is why so many people are drawn to her. It's remarkable to observe. She's this unique combination of someone super gifted and driven with this inviting, fun-loving spirit. As a result, Carrie has always had a large circle of friends. As she should. She is definitely someone you want to be around.

GBS – The Immovable Object.

Like any good story, we, too, must have a villain. For this journey, as you know, the villain is GBS. And quite a formidable one at that. Ever the overachiever, Carrie didn't just have a typical case of GBS. She had about the worst version possible. And secondary complications on top, just for good measure. Carrie doesn't do anything small and this lifelong trend held for GBS.

So, we have an unstoppable force and an immovable object (the pun— since GBS causes paralysis—is somewhat intended. We all like good puns, right?). Unsurprisingly, I'm going to tell you that the unstoppable force triumphs over the immovable object. Not because I have the benefit of hindsight and that's what happened. I bring this up now because this is how I knew when Carrie got sick that she was going to come out of it just fine, if not better than fine. I knew this with every fiber of my being. I never had any doubts. Truly. (Although, had I been told at the time that Carrie's rehabilitation physicians thought she might never get off her ventilator, I might have had some doubts. Fortunately, I didn't learn that until this whole chapter was well behind her.) I believe in science, so I knew if the doctors could stop the ascending paralysis, the rest of the story— the recovery—was up to Carrie. And, Carrie being Carrie, would put all her focus on recovery and would smash all expectations along the way. And that's exactly what she did. As an unstoppable force, there's nothing that Carrie cannot do. We just needed the GBS to stop its progression and then Carrie would do what she's done her entire life – come out on top. Kicking ass is pretty much the only thing she knows how to do. I love and admire her for it.

The Early Days

Heartbreaking. That's really the only way to describe the time Carrie spent at the neurological ICU at Northwestern. Remember when I said that Carrie's GBS was the worst possible version? Not only was the medical situation awful (and trust me, it was), the timing of the illness coincided with Carrie's birthday and Christmas. Sure, when your birthday is a week before Christmas, and you contract something as serious as GBS, that's bound to happen. But, in what scenario should anyone have to spend her thirty-sixth birthday AND Christmas in the Neuro ICU? So, like I said, heartbreaking.

What made the early weeks of her illness so troubling is that this is the time when we effectively, albeit temporarily, "lost" Carrie. She was intubated so she couldn't talk. Not only that, but the tubes and such covered most of her face. She was also in an incredible amount of pain. To combat the pain, she was on what seemed a healthy Fentanyl drip. Healthy because she was asleep a lot, which I imagine was for the best. But, the combination of the narcotics and intubation meant that when Carrie was awake, it wasn't really her. There was no vibrancy in her eyes. No shine. No spark to give any inclination that our

Carrie was still there, biding her time until she could show GBS who was the boss. But I know that's what she was doing.

Fortunately, the ICU doctors were able to stop the ascending paralysis. That was an extraordinarily shiny day. However, the paralysis had reached her chest, so she could not move any of her limbs. Nor did she have the strength to breathe on her own, so the intubation was swapped out for a tracheostomy and the ventilator was to be a co-lead in this story. The road to recovery was going to be long. It turns out, nerves don't regenerate very quickly in the human body.

The neuro ICU wasn't without its light-hearted moments, making the best of a bad situation and all. Due to the trach, Carrie couldn't talk. Because no one in her support village was any good at reading lips, at least not at that point, a speech therapist provided us an alphabet chart to help us communicate more effectively. We'd ask Carrie which row the letter she wanted was on (e.g., one, two, three, etc.), then count over the letters in the row until you got to the right one. As you can imagine, this was not the quickest way to communicate. Once Carrie would provide the first few letters, everyone would start guessing what she was trying to say or ask as there were definitely trends in her requests, comments, and questions. However, we had a bit of wrinkle in the process. Despite her long list of qualities, Carrie is not a good speller and she was still pretty heavily medicated (both pain medication and Propofol as she had a significant amount of anxiety). These circumstances combined for some interesting "conversations" with Carrie.

One day in particular, I was spending time with Carrie and her Dad. She wanted to tell us something, so we pulled out the alphabet board. I had heard that Dick, Carrie's wonderful father, was not the best at running the alphabet board, so I stepped up to try my hand. Carrie had identified three to five letters, which made absolutely no sense. They weren't the beginning of any known word. (Oftentimes Carrie would doze off during spelling, losing her mental place and duplicating or skipping letters, or maybe she was just frustrated by our lousy board communication skills.) Dick and I must have suggested aardvark or armadillo half a dozen times. Because when you're paralyzed, and in the ICU, you want to talk about random animals. Eventually, we figured out that she was trying to spell hallucinating. As in the Propofol was making her hallucinate. We felt a bit of achievement when we solved that riddle, but then had to solve the mystery of the hallucinations. That happened a lot with Carrie's GBS; a win followed by an unexpected wrinkle.

Epitome of Carrie in the ICU? On December 20th, she told me to write down the following question to ask the doctors during rounds the next morning: "What else can I be doing to progress faster?" She still had nearly a week remaining in the ICU and months in rehab, but, as I had expected, she was ready to show GBS who was boss.

Winding Road of Rehabilitation

The Rehabilitation Institute of Chicago (RIC, now the Shirly Ryan AbilityLab) is one of the heroes of this story. That place is amazing. The staff are exceptional. And, for Carrie, the respiratory therapists were truly lifesavers. The speech therapists literally brought me to tears because they taught Carrie to speak with her talking trach. With a talking trach, you have to speak while inhaling; normally, we exhale while we speak. She had to learn to talk "backwards"! In one speech therapy session I observed, as she was building strength and putting more and more words together, she told me, "Will (her three-and-a-half-year-old son) is coming tomorrow. I want to tell him I love him and miss him." That was an incredible moment that I was thrilled to experience.

But it was daunting to get a sense of all the things Carrie had to relearn. Sitting up. Swallowing. Moving/controlling fingers. Walking. Talking. She had to relearn the movements, with each task having many subparts, and then build strength. For every single task. It's no wonder it took three months. And yet incredible that it only took three months.

At RIC, Carrie was ALWAYS hot. Not just warm, HOT. So much so that we'd have to fill bags full of ice and put them around her to cool her off. Apparently, regenerating nerves throws multiple body systems out of whack. I also remember her regular requests for massages. Between the nerve re-growth and intense physical and occupational therapy, Carrie was sore much of the time. I'd massage her multiple times a night if she wanted. Shoulders, arms, hands, fingers, legs, feet. And now she knows how the people in her life rank in terms of massage skills. I hear I'm towards the top of the list.

Epitome of Carrie at RIC? She was hands down a staff favorite. This is no exaggeration. Since her discharge from RIC, she has added many of her RIC care team as Facebook friends. As I said, people are drawn to her.

The F**king Delicate Flower

For the most part, Carrie's recovery was a straight line. Given her age and fitness, she was able to surpass expectations for her physical, occupational, and speech therapy. On those fronts, she was truly a rock star. Pretty much from her first week at RIC, she was highly motivated, focused, and would get upset when her daily schedule did not include therapy appointments with all three disciplines. She always wanted to know what she could be doing to recover faster. That's true for everything except Carrie's windpipe and pulmonary function. As we would discover, repeatedly, Carrie's windpipe is a delicate flower.

I'm sure Carrie and others will go into all the specific issues with her windpipe, but suffice it to say, it was the source of all the twists, turns, hurdles, challenges, and backtracking of her recovery. Who knew four inches of tissue could cause so much grief? She was off the vent. Then back on the vent. There were surgeries and procedures. After one surgery, when she had part of her windpipe removed, her chin was actually stitched to her chest for several days. Can you even imagine? So uncomfortable! Then after one of her windpipe surgeries her incision got infected. Everything with her damn windpipe was a mess.

On the days that Carrie got down, it was typically because of her windpipe. Makes total sense; we all love talking and eating. But even if her spirits got down, they never stayed down for long. And, in the end, she got off the ventilator for good and her windpipe healed. That's just the kind of girl she is. An unstoppable force who beat an immovable object.

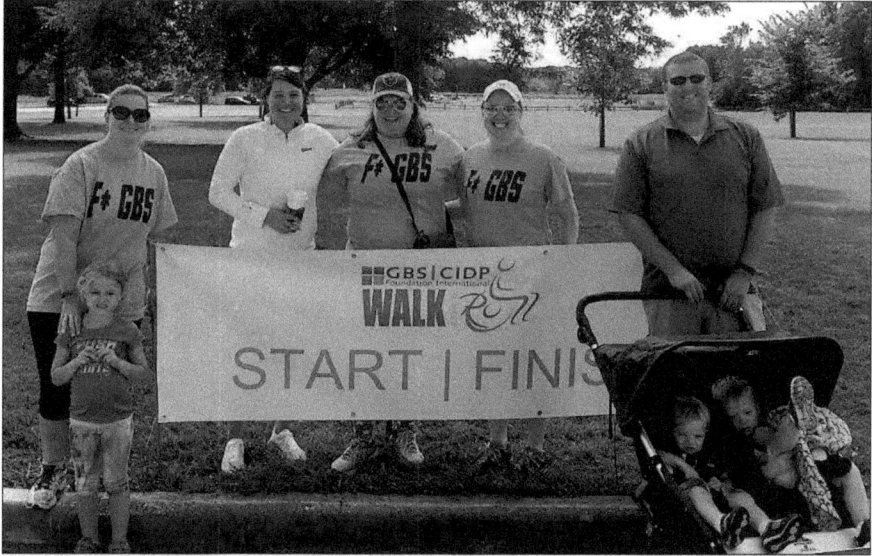

Carrie with her friends Laura (and family), Jennifer, and Brooke doing a walk benefitting the GBS Foundation.

From Patty Carmichael
Carrie's Best Friend

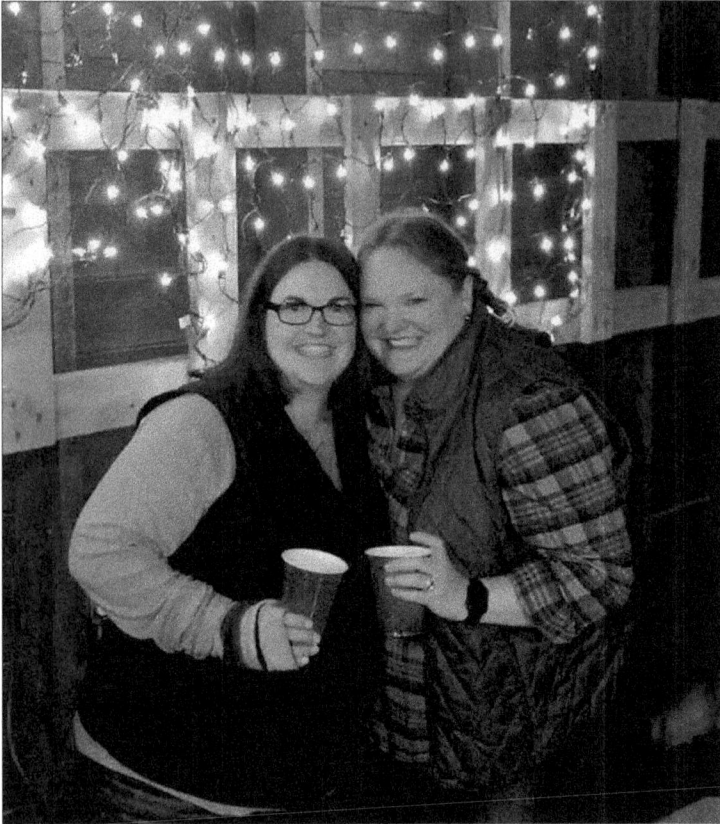

Carrie and best friend Patty.

Patty text: When am I going to get to catch up with you again?

Carrie text: Patty, it's Jeff. Carrie is not good. It might be a while before you can talk to her.

Patty text: OK, tell her I'm thinking of her.

The exact series of events escapes me. However, I remember where I was sitting in my house when I was texting with Laura Ball. I was asking her how serious Carrie's condition was and if she thought I should drive to Chicago. Never in my life had I wanted to be in Chicago more than that moment. Laura told me to hold off and not come yet. They were doing everything they could and we had to just wait.

"She's going to make it through this though, right?" I hesitantly asked. Then the tears, the worry, and the prayers continued and intensified. I constantly debated with myself and Todd if I should drive to Chicago because even though I couldn't do anything, I would at least be closer.

We were told Carrie was being moved from the suburbs to downtown and intubated. I felt I had to do something, and I finally decided to go visit Carrie on her birthday, December 18, 2013. I had brought paper crowns for us all to color and wear in celebration. I had reached out to friends and family to send birthday wishes along with selfies. I was planning to read them to Carrie throughout the day. I was ready for what I thought would be an upbeat reunion to celebrate her birthday even though she was in the hospital.

Holy shit. I was not prepared for walking into Carrie's ICU room. She needed all the strength we could give. It wasn't a time to be shocked or scared because that's what she was going through, but I didn't quite comprehend that yet. My best friend lying on a hospital bed with tubes down her throat and up her nose. Not moving. I don't think we quite got through all the birthday wishes that day. Come to find out later, Carrie was having a really shitty day. Not necessarily a birthday she'll want to remember.

People seemed to be in constant motion around her room. Her parents and Jeff were there, and Carrie was trying to communicate with them by moving her eyes to different letters on a board. Dick wanted to finish what he thought she was trying to say. "Trying," being the key word. He wasn't always correct, but we had to learn a new way of communication which served to be frustrating on all sides. One of the many doctors came in and asked Carrie if she wanted to have the tubes removed and replaced with a trach and feeding tube. She ferociously communicated Y-E-S. There was no hesitation and I think that shocked most of us at the time. Why couldn't they figure out what was going on and how to make Carrie better...now! In a world of instant gratification we couldn't understand how many hours, months, years it would actually take once they figured it out. In that moment, Carrie wanted the tubes out! Who knew in this whole process we would find out how delicate her windpipe is?

Jeff's parents brought Will to see Carrie and he lit up her eyes! She really wanted him to sit on her lap, and I could tell he really wanted to help Carrie and make her better. More and more questions, fewer and fewer answers.

Kathy Lunzmann flew in that day as well. Ardie and Greg (Jeff's parents) had colds so, as a precaution, they wore masks before they came into Carrie's room. There were a lot of smiles and a lot of love in that room that day. That was what we could give Carrie at the time. The fear was definitely lingering, but never mentioned. A few friends from Carrie's work came to visit, and I don't think anyone could imagine that scene without actually witnessing it for themselves. I will see it in my mind forever. Every single person gave Carrie strength when they saw her, and immediately broke down just outside the room. It's extremely difficult to see such a strong person incapacitated. We all felt helpless and craved to do more for Carrie.

I came back on January 18th, and Carrie was no longer in ICU. She couldn't talk but was still communicating through slight movements and her eyes. Those eyes were alive with passion and hope. Stephanie Anderson and I came up to visit a few weeks later and I was able to take a shift and spend the night. It may have been January or February, I'm not sure, but it was COLD. Since Carrie's nerves were regaining feeling, she was always HOT! I slept with my winter coat on, but I didn't care because I could actually be there to help.

My next memory was the day—yes, I should remember the date and time—when I was driving home from work and it was snowing out. I know exactly where I was when my cell phone rang. I looked and Carrie was calling me. I wasn't going to turn down that phone call. I picked up and heard her say my name in a very soft scratchy voice. It was amazing! Her mom was there with her, helping translate. I still get emotional thinking about it. We didn't talk for long. I hung up the phone, pulled my car over, and burst into tears. Carrie was talking! What an amazing accomplishment!

I was lucky the next time I visited at the RIC; it was the few hours they let Carrie practice talking. It would wear her out, but I wanted to just sit and listen to her. I was awestruck by how well Carrie was progressing. She had good and bad days, but she never gave up.

I am so lucky and honored to have Carrie in my life. She has so many who support and love her. There's not one of us that wouldn't have switched places with her, even for a minute to give her a break during her diagnosis and recovery. I can't imagine all she had to go through and wish I could have covered more shifts. To say she inspires me is an understatement.

It's difficult to write this and remember back because Carrie has made a full or very close to full recovery. She had a miracle in Zach and is back to living life to the fullest every day with her family. I know she is still scared sometimes when she gets sick, but I'm proud of her every day for her determination and positive outlook. It's contagious and takes me out of my comfort zone most of the time.

Thank you, Carrie, for being my friend, showing me what living life to the fullest looks like, and having the strength every day to learn and move forward from this incapacitating disease. You told GBS to f**k off and you won. We all won. Love you!

From Ardie Grimes
Carrie's Mother-in-law

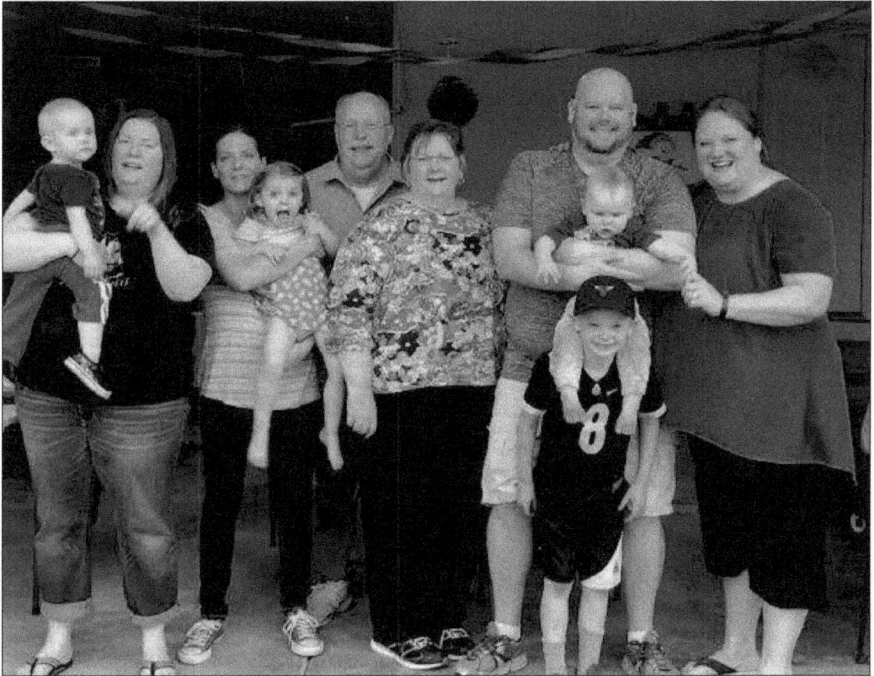

Grimes Family: Zeph, Lynette, Charise (Jeff's sisters), Ella, Greg, Ardie, Jeff, Zach, Will, and Carrie.

Our perspective of Carrie's GBS journey

Our first clue that something was happening was a phone call on Sunday, December 8th, from our son, Jeff, who told us that Carrie was in the hospital, and the physicians didn't know what was wrong. We could hear so much worry and stress in his voice and promised him that we would be praying. We also told him that since Greg was retired, we could come up to Libertyville and help out at any time. Since Dick and Kathy (Carrie's parents) had gone up immediately, Jeff didn't think that we needed to come right away.

I remember calling my sister, Beth, who is a nurse, telling her about Carrie and asking her to pray. We both thought at the time that it was Guillain-Barré Syndrome, because we had a family friend who had it several years ago. Beth kept calling or texting me, asking if they had started treatment yet. Each time, I had to say, "No, they are still doing tests." Finally, Jeff let us know that the neurologist was "almost positive" that she had GBS. By Thursday three IVIG treatments had been given but were not helping much. Jeff's phone calls and emails kept getting scarier: Carrie had to be intubated and was not able to talk; the weakness is progressing upwards; the IVIG is apparently not working. So, the decision was made to transfer Carrie from Northwestern Memorial hospital in Lake Forest to the downtown Chicago Northwestern Memorial hospital. Subsequently, we left home on Saturday to drive to Chicago. We arrived on the 15th. Carrie had the first plasmapheresis treatment on Monday, making her extremely tired and achy.

After arriving in Libertyville, our role was primarily to keep the home fires burning and do whatever we could to support Jeff and Will, and by extension, Carrie. We took Will to school and picked him up, attempting to maintain his normal schedule. I cooked, did laundry, and cleaned as I worried and prayed about what was going on at the hospital. Greg was the chauffeur and early morning on-call person, getting up when Will did and giving him breakfast. He also spent many hours in the basement rough-housing and playing ball with Will.

With us staying at the house, Jeff was able to spend more hours at the hospital with Carrie, though he drove home every couple of days to spend some time with Will, sleep in his own bed, de-compress a bit and pick up some clean clothes. It was important for Jeff to have us there to talk to; to express fears and frustrations. We listened, encouraged, hugged and served him; then we prayed fervently, and later, I cried.

Will, being only three years old, knew that Mommy was in the hospital so the doctors could take care of her. When visiting in the ICU, it was pretty intimidating for him when Mommy couldn't talk like she normally could; it was difficult for him to even snuggle with her with so many tubes, IVs, etc. Jeff would pick him up and "fly" him up to kiss Carrie, and her eyes would light up as she enjoyed the kiss.

On December 18th, Greg and I picked up Carrie's birthday cake (that Jeff had ordered weeks before) from the bakery in Libertyville and delivered it to her room in ICU. Will was able to see Mommy, and so many of her friends, for a very short time, but Carrie's second plasmapheresis treatment was started that afternoon, cutting short the visit.

Dick, Kathy, and Andy drove back up to Libertyville to spend time with Carrie over the Christmas holiday, so we drove home on Monday, December 23rd. We drove home, and then up to Lincoln, Nebraska, to have our Christmas with Charise and Brian, our daughter and son-in-law and Lynette, our other daughter.

Meanwhile, on December 26th, Carrie was discharged from the ICU and moved to the Rehab Institute of Chicago. We drove back to Libertyville, breaking up the trip with an overnight stay in Springfield because of snow and ice on the roads.

We tried to keep Jeff and Carrie up to date on what was happening at their home and with Will. One night, while I was bathing him, he said to me, "I am special, and Mom and Dad are special, but you and Grandad are not special, 'cause you are OLD!" We continued Carrie's practice of sending a "Daily Will," a photo and short excerpt of something that happened to Will that day. After we upgraded to smart phones (and figured out how to use them!), we were able to also send videos of Will's activities and antics.

Then, with Greg needing to pay bills, do the income taxes and catch up a bit on stuff at home, we brought Will home to Baldwin City with us on January 20th. He was a trooper on the trip – we bought a new Berenstain Bears DVD and he watched it six times on the trip, along with playing Magna-Tiles and reading lots of books. Only once did he say, "Gram, I think this is a really long trip!" While Will was here, we went to open gym at gymnastics, went to the children's museum in Kansas City, went to the library to get books, played with trains, and hung out with Aunt Lynette.

On January 24th, we took Will to Lincoln to stay with Dick, Kathy and Andy for a few days. Our daughter, Charise was expecting our first granddaughter, but she wanted to snuggle longer with her Mommy, and did not arrive on her due date, so we came back home, and returned to Lincoln after Ella's birth on January 27th. We stayed with Charise and Brian and got to meet Ella and hold her lots. Due to another storm, we delayed our trip back to Libertyville until February 7th. Will was SO glad to see his Daddy that evening and was more excited to see Mommy a couple of days later— his first trip to the Rehab Institute.

Trips to the Rehab hospital were challenging. Greg absolutely hates driving in downtown Chicago traffic, so he would be irritable on those days. Will often acted out on those days, especially when leaving the hospital. One day, I asked Jeff to walk with us to the elevator to say goodbye to Will. As the elevator doors closed, Will started sobbing and cried all the way down to the ground level. He fell on the floor in the lobby, and was crying inconsolably. I finally managed to pick him up, sans coat, and carried him out to the car and got him into the car seat; the poor guy was just a limp, sobbing bundle of hurt. Jeff said later that he could hear Will all the way down the elevator until we got off. So we learned that having Jeff come down to the lobby, put him in the car seat, and start the DVD player to distract him worked much better when it came time to leave.

When we visited the Rehab hospital, Greg and I tried to wander off and give Carrie, Jeff, and Will as much family time as possible. That was the primary reason for bringing Will to visit, and we didn't want to interrupt that precious time. The more times Will visited, and the more progress Carrie made, the visits became easier. I tried to take along a few things they could play together. Matchbox cars and trains were popular. Later on, we discovered games in the family lounge. It was a red-letter day when we walked into Carrie's room and she was able to lift her hand and wave at us! When Will tired of talking to Mom, and needed something quiet to do, the iPad was always available, and he would sit on Carrie's bed, snuggled between her legs and watch movies or programs.

Will had lots of fun playing outside in all the snow in February and March, even though it was so cold. There were HUGE dirty piles of snow all around the center of the cul-de-sac where their house is. He enjoyed the challenge of climbing up and peeking over the top. Some of the older neighbor kids had created a slide on one side and he had fun sliding down that. He also liked using his new "diggers" to move the snow around like Uncle Andy. Inside, Will and I played with Play-Doh a lot and he learned to play Go Fish. Because it seemed like winter dragged on for so long, Jeff ordered a small trampoline for Will to use inside. It really did help him expend some of his energy. On the day the aluminum ramp was installed, Will spent about an hour poking tiny pieces of feather grass in many of the holes in the ramp. Then he rolled the basketball down the ramp and tried riding his bike down it, too. I think Will used the ramp more than Carrie did!

Carrie came home on Wednesday, April 2nd, able to walk up the temporary ramp, and manage the stairs. We stayed a few more weeks until Kathy was finished with her senatorial duties and was able to stay with Carrie, Jeff, and Will. We left Libertyville on Saturday April 19th, to spend the Easter weekend with Charise and Brian before returning home to Baldwin City.

Though the circumstances were far from ideal, we were privileged to spend such extended time with Will, getting to know him so much better than just a weekend visit several times a year. I think we have an extra special bond with him because of the amount of time we spent together and hope that we can continue to nourish and maintain that special relationship.

We are so very, very proud of Jeff and the way he responded during this life crisis. His first thought was always for Carrie, and what he could do to make things easier or better for her. He kept everyone updated with progress reports; scheduled friends and family to stay with Carrie at the hospital when he could not be there; demonstrated how to use the letter board to communicate with her; helped us with suggestions for dealing with a three-year-old; still managed to work online from Carrie's hospital room; and so many other things. His next concern was for Will, that he maintained a somewhat normal schedule. He ensured that Will had play time with Dad when he was home. Jeff was often physically and emotionally exhausted, but still put Carrie's and Will's needs before his own. He probably wanted to smack me when I started telling him that he needed to take care of himself, too; that he could not afford to get sick and not be able to spend time with Carrie.

Before this turns into a book, I have to mention all of Carrie's friends who brought meals to the house for us while she was in the hospital and also after her return home. We really appreciated all those yummy meals, but I vow to never take lasagna to a sick friend ever again. We had an excess of lasagna, especially since I made several pans of it and put them in the freezer! A special thanks to Meg who brought me her Mom's homemade chicken soup when I was sick with the crud and had nearly lost my voice.

From Greg Grimes
Carrie's Father-in-law

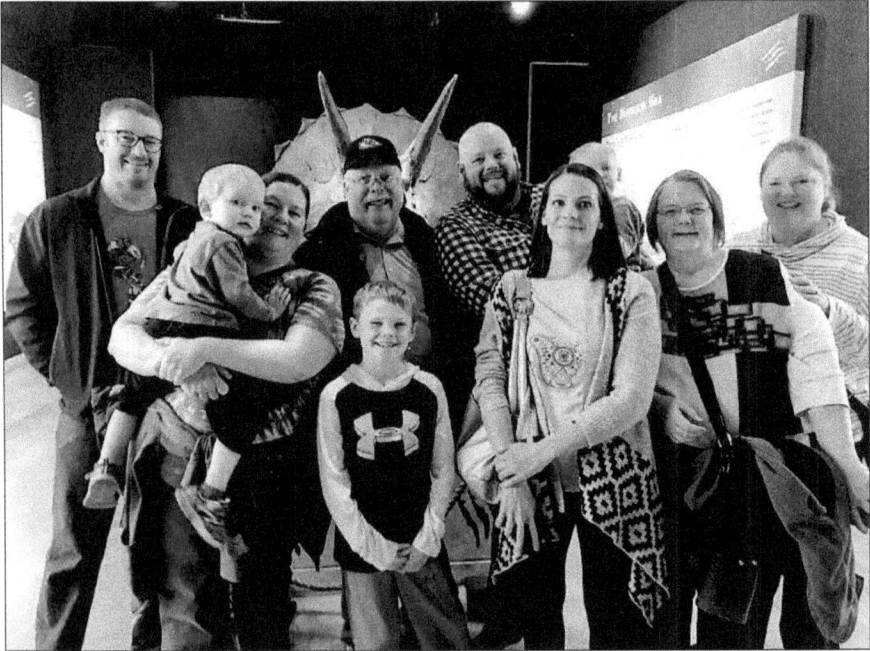

Members of the Grimes family: Brophy, Zeph, Lynette, Greg, Will, Jeff, Charise, Zach, Ardie and Carrie.

After delaying way too long, I will add my comments and perspective, even though Ardie has covered pretty much everything we experienced with Carrie's fight with GBS. Ardie's recall of dates is much better than mine.

I recall Jeff's first phone call and the worry and stress in his voice when he called to tell us about Carrie's illness in December 2013. I did not realize how serious this illness was at first. Jeff asked us to pray for Carrie and him, which of course we did and asked our church and family to pray.

I had retired in May 2013, so we had time and it worked out for us to be able to travel to Libertyville when Jeff asked us to come and take care of Will. I recall when we started driving from Kansas and through Missouri, it was raining with the temperature hovering right at 32 degrees. Not a fun travel day, but of course, nothing compared to what Carrie was going through.

As Ardie said, we tried to keep Will on his regular schedule as much as possible. I know Will missed his Mom and Dad very much, since they were both gone from home. And as Ardie said, Will was very distraught whenever we left after a visit to RIC, or whenever Jeff came home and then had to go back to downtown Chicago.

I recall Will being very hesitant to get close to Carrie in the hospital at first, when she had all the tubes, and he didn't understand why Mom could not talk to him.

I remember all the snow and the cold "Chiberia" winter months that we spent at Jeff and Carrie's house caring for Will. That was one of the coldest and snowiest winters on record for Chicago. Will loved being able to climb and play on the snow pile out in the middle of the cul-de-sac.

I recall Jeff's fears that he might lose Carrie. I also remember his concern of losing the house that they had just purchased that year and how he would raise Will. We tried to reassure him, but not sure how much we did.

I am very proud of Jeff for how he supported Carrie and cared for her through all of her ordeal in fighting GBS. How he stayed with her in the hospital for so many days and nights is amazing and a testimony of his love for her.

I am proud of Carrie for her strong efforts in recovering from GBS. I give thanks to the Lord daily for answered prayers for Carrie's healing and recovery from GBS. I am also thankful for the doctors and all medical staff that helped Carrie in her recovery.

I Corinthians 13:7 (love) "bears all things, believes all things, hopes all things, endures all things." V.13, "And now abide faith, hope, love, these three, but the greatest of these is love."

Ecclesiastes 4:9, 10: "Two are better than one.... For if either of them falls, the one will lift up his companion."

From Andy Campbell
Carrie's Brother

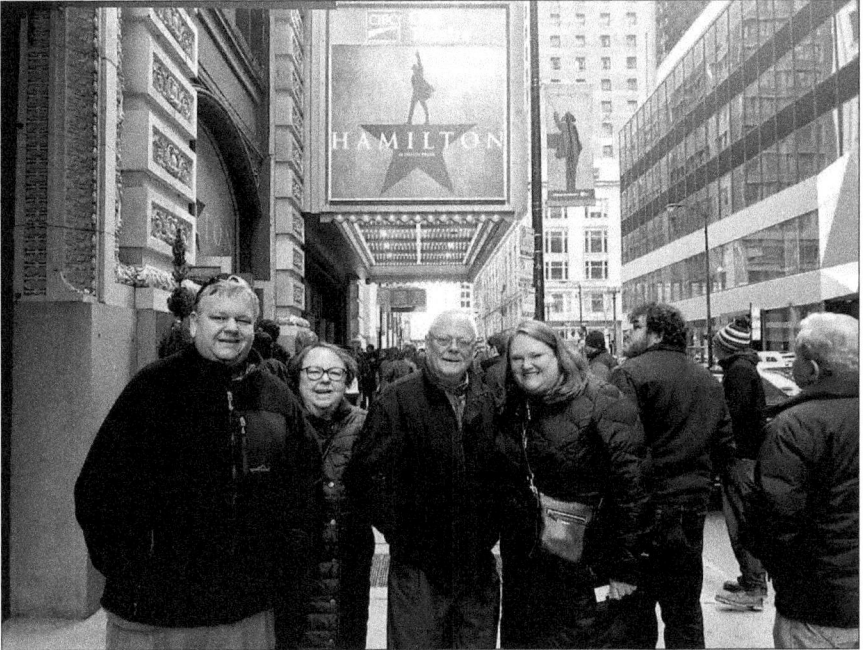

Carrie with her brother, Mom, and Dad.

As a big brother, you learn early on that you have a tough job. On one hand, you have a born "enemy" in a little sister. She's always stealing your toys, complaining to Mom that you won't let her watch what she wants on TV, and repeatedly finding new and ever imaginative ways to get on your nerves. The other side, though, is the side where you put all of that aside, as it is your job to protect your little sister from the world. Whether it is someone picking on her, her choice in men to date, or simply being supportive when things get tough, as a big brother, you put the tension and battles between you on the shelf and you do what you can to protect your little sister. When it comes to something like GBS, however, there isn't a bully to intimidate, a date to scare, or a battle to fight. What does a big brother do when his sister is fighting something like GBS?

When I first heard that Carrie had been hospitalized with GBS it didn't mean much. She and her family had been home to Lincoln for Thanksgiving a week or so previously and she'd seemed fine; well, as fine as someone coming down with a cold can be. She, Jeff, and I had participated in the first ever Campbell Family Turkey Trot. More than fifty extended family and friends had braved near zero-degree temperatures to walk or run a Thanksgiving 5k run. While I came in last of those who ran the full distance, I was pretty proud to finish the race—partially because of the weather but also as the football-lineman size guy in the family.

I mention this because I was a bit happier than I should admit that Carrie and her husband Jeff had dropped out shortly into the race. Both were fighting colds and Carrie was actually coughing so badly she was coughing up some blood. At the time, she didn't seem any different to me than anyone with a chest cold coming on. She slept a bit more, let the rest of us dote on Nephew Will to take some stress off her and Jeff, and did what all of us do when we catch a cold. She drank her fluids, popped some meds, and seemed to resign herself to having a cold to fight off as she returned to Chicago after the holiday. When they left, Carrie seemed a bit off, but the cold didn't seem that bad to me and I put it out of my head. Everyone gets a cold here or there during the winter. This wouldn't be anything serious to worry about.

As life moved from Thanksgiving to preparing for Christmas, my life was busy. Our family nursery and landscape company was busy installing Christmas lights, maintenance crews were trying to complete fall landscape cleanups, and we were still trying to complete some last landscape installations before Mother Nature shut us down for the winter. As the manager of our installation and maintenance department, I was busy trying to help get as much accomplished as I could. My sister and her health slipped out of my mind as I focused on everything else. At least until I received a call from my mother, I think on a Monday. I remember her telling me that Carrie had gotten sick and was in the hospital. I don't remember whether the words Guillain-Barré syndrome were mentioned in the first call. What I do remember is Mom mentioning something about Carrie losing feeling in her legs and being unsteady on her feet over the weekend, so they had gone to the emergency room. The docs thought she was simply dehydrated from her cold and so they gave her an IV and sent her home. I remember being told that after another day or so, she was so unsteady on her feet that she had to slide down the stairs on her butt to get back to the hospital. I remember being worried because this was my little sister and I couldn't do anything about it.

Carrie Campbell Grimes

That first phone call was Mom telling me she and Dad were leaving for Chicago and that hopefully it wouldn't be as serious as it sounded. She told me that Carrie had begun losing control and feeling in her legs and arms and it was time to get to Chicago to help and be there for Carrie. I remember sitting at my work desk thinking that things were bad, but it wouldn't be too bad; a few days in the hospital, some medication once they knew what was going on, and Carrie would put this thing behind her. Little did I know then what Carrie would have to endure to recover from this thing called GBS.

During that first week, my life was more normal compared to the rest of the family. I couldn't do much from Nebraska, but I did what I could to support my parents and kept busy with work. We're used to being busy with our family business during the holidays, so while I talked to my parents almost daily, Carrie's fight seemed like something distant. I could picture what she was going through and deep down it did scare me, but this was my sister—the hard charging athlete; the type-A personality who sometimes overscheduled our family trips when we went to Chicago to visit; a woman who never seemed to shirk from a challenge. Our parents did what they could to keep me updated on what was happening, but what could I do beyond support those helping her and send thoughts and prayers her direction?

As the days passed and I did more research into GBS, I could tell this was not as simple as many other health issues she could be facing. Not to belittle anyone facing cancer or diabetes, or any of a dozen other life-altering issues, but GBS seemed so different to me. It is a syndrome versus a disease because they really don't know what causes it. It is a medical issue without real specific drugs to treat it. Since GBS causes

292

your own immune system to attack your own body, it can be different for each patient. As a person who likes to know more about something I don't understand, the more I read, the more GBS seemed like something out of a science fiction novel. And, for the life of me, I couldn't quite picture my sister going through it. I had no pictures, no firsthand knowledge of what GBS was doing to Carrie. So while I worried, and while I did what I could from afar, it all seemed so unreal. I don't think I ever got my mind around the fact that GBS could kill her. I had read the statistics, so I knew there was a chance, but not seeing her in the hospital kept me insulated from reality. On some levels, I wonder if how I thought about her struggle those first weeks would be different if I had made that trip with my parents.

As the days passed and we realized this was not going to be something Carrie fought off quickly, our family began to make changes in our plans for Christmas. Originally, the plan had been for Carrie and her family to join us in Lincoln for Christmas. Jeff has a sister who lives here with her family and hosts their side of the family for Christmas. Both Carrie's and Jeff's families would be in Lincoln, making celebrations easier. GBS had other plans for us. My parents would return to Lincoln to handle some things then we would drive back up to Chicago to spend Christmas and New Year's doing our best to help with Will, assist Carrie in the hospital, and to try to celebrate the holidays.

It would be one of a few times I had been away from my job for more than a week and my longest visit to relatives. We stayed so long we ended up doing laundry. In fact, when we left Nebraska our return date was up in the air. Of course, little things like that were easy to deal with compared to what Carrie was going through.

As we prepared for our trip, my feelings for what Carrie was going through became more real. Knowing that we would visit and see her was both good and bad for me. On the good side, I would physically be there for her. Even though we couldn't do anything, just knowing that I would physically be near felt as if I were doing something. The bad side was knowing I would have to face this evil thing attacking my sister. I will admit it scared me. It's like the stories that extreme sport athletes like NASCAR drivers don't go to funerals so they won't be reminded of how dangerous their sport can be to them. By not being there physically, I could remain in a bit of denial. This wasn't as bad as everyone was saying; my sister wasn't in a hospital bed unable to move. GBS hadn't put her on a ventilator needing help to breathe. She wouldn't have to stay there for weeks and months to come. Denial was a place I could explore even though my logical side knew all of the above, and more, were true and my sister wasn't in a good place with GBS.

As I went to visit Carrie for the first time, I told myself, just as I had been from the start of this GBS bullshit, my job was to support everyone else. I knew I would be able to help by helping others. Whether it would be to help with Will, run errands or make dinner while Mom and Dad went to sit with Carrie for the day, or whatever else needed to be done. This mindset allowed me to still keep one foot in denial.

As many do, I have used and do use humor as a way to push back at difficult situations. Carrie has since given me grief that when I first walked in to see her, I cracked a joke. Yep, I did. I told her that if she really wanted us to come to Chicago for

Christmas, all she had to do was ask. While she is right that I crack jokes instead of being emotional (I could have gotten emotional when I first saw her; I did inside.) I quickly realized that everyone else was being emotional. Whether it was the right or wrong move I felt that I would try to lighten the mood, or try to offer an alternative type of support. Maybe that is the guys way of dealing with difficult situations.

Cracking jokes or giving each other some grief was the way Carrie and I dealt with each other growing up. On some level, I felt that if I treated her differently than I had for years, it would somehow add to her worry. I thought that her seeing me being emotional or too nice about her fight with GBS would end up adding to her challenge. If I treated her too nicely, she might think I knew something and should be worried. So, I decided to treat her nicely and to help when possible but without being too emotional or too nice. There were others around her who seemed to be emotionally involved so I would be the one to take a step back toward what I saw as normal.

As we moved past that first visit, it became easier and easier for me to fall into a rhythm and move out of denial. I probably went through what so many do when dealing with a loved one fighting something like GBS. I could now physically witness Carrie's fight. I could experience it. I could understand it. Each visit, each experience, helped me come to grips with what she was going through. I saw how I could leave denial behind and truly be there to help her and the rest of the family—with humor and other types of support.

GBS is a horrible thing for anyone to experience but, as with so many other things in life, it can be rough for the family trying to support the person going through GBS—especially for a spouse. I'm not sure I could have done what Carrie's husband Jeff did during her long recovery. His challenge of balancing his work, trying to keep home life as normal as possible, and supporting Carrie through it all was amazing to see. The man deserves a medal. I don't know Jeff well enough to say he is an extroverted introvert like me, but I know we both need our down time. I would describe this as time when I'm not being pressured by life, work, or anyone else; time I can do something for me and not have to worry about the big picture. Whether that is how Jeff would describe it, I don't know. If you are any type of introvert, you know exactly what I mean. What I do know is that everything I saw Jeff doing for my sister and my nephew couldn't have left him much down time. I know he must have taken time for himself as Carrie fought GBS, but it definitely wasn't as much as he probably needed.

After we arrived in Chicago for the holidays, life settled into a rough rhythm. Many days our job was to focus on taking care of Will. No one really does as good a job as a parent, but we did our best to keep the little guy heading in the right direction. Sometimes that meant getting him up, feeding him breakfast, and getting him off to school. Other times that meant cooking the dinner he asked for then making something else when he changed his mind. Many parents would not be so accommodating as it happens, but as the uncle and grandparents of a child missing his mother because of GBS, we compromised a lot. While there were times Will was out of sorts, or would ask questions about his mom in the hospital, most of the time I was amazed at how well he dealt with the whole GBS experience. Maybe young kids are more resilient. Will certainly seemed to be.

We did our best to try to make Christmas as normal as possible for Will. We made Chex mix, letting him help count out the ingredients. We took over placing the Elf on the Shelf in new locations each day for Will to find, including on Christmas Eve when the Elf found his way to the top of the Christmas tree hanging from the star. As we drove him to and from school, we looked at the Christmas lights. While Carrie and Jeff worried about GBS, we tried to keep things as normal as possible for Will. While I think we succeeded in some ways, it wasn't the same because we were doing it without Carrie and Jeff.

As Christmas arrived, we did what we could with our iPhones and iPads to FaceTime so Carrie and Jeff could experience Will opening his presents. We handled all of the "Some Assembly Required" projects for Santa. Any parent knows how much fun that assembly can be. We let Will help everyone else open their presents. A three-year-old believes every present under the tree was meant for him. As he peeled off the wrapping paper, I asked Will what he thought a present might be. He would simply look at me and reply, "It's a box. I don't know what it is Uncle Andy."

As much as we tried to celebrate Christmas as if it was any other year, it just wasn't truly Christmas. My parents, Will and I opened presents and did our family traditions like having our standard egg dish Christmas morning, eating some pickled herring, and listening to Christmas music. We did what we could to make Christmas be Christmas, but something was definitely missing. We went through the motions, but it never seemed quite right. Without Carrie and Jeff with us at home, Christmas seemed hollow. We didn't have a choice. GBS had taken normal away from us as we tried to have a normal

Christmas for Will. It's not fair to take away Christmas from a three-year-old.

We definitely had a white Christmas in Chicago. In fact, I think it snowed something like twenty-five inches over the couple of weeks we were there. The pile of snow in the cul-de-sac where Carrie and Jeff live was so high that it dwarfed Will and came up to about my chest. Most days we had some fun bundling Will up to go play in the snow, allowing him to crawl all over the pile.

As we moved from Christmas onto New Year's some of our thoughts beyond Carrie turned to football, the bowl games, and our beloved Nebraska Cornhuskers playing in the Gator Bowl on New Year's Day. I can say that since I was a young child, I have never missed watching a Husker Bowl game, but this one will be stuck in my memory because of how we experienced the game. During our time in Chicago, we tried to get Will down to see Carrie at least once or twice a week. We had decided we would take Will down to see Carrie on New Year's Day. Our plan was to leave early, arrive before the game started, watch the game with Carrie in her room, then return home. As some would say, the best laid plans.

Beginning New Year's Eve night and continuing well into New Year's Day, Chicago experienced another snowstorm bringing with it ten to fourteen inches of new snow. Our plan to leave early had to be pushed to allow time for the snow plows to work on the roads. We were okay though, because I had realized a few days prior that Mom's satellite radio did not get any sports stations, so I had paid for an app to stream the radio broadcast of the game. We would just listen to the game as we drove to the hospital and watch the rest of the game with Carrie. We ended up leaving late, driving through the snowstorm on highways seemingly barely touched by the snowplows, thinking we might get stuck at any time—while trying to listen to the game. The drive that normally took an hour took more than two to two-and-a-half hours. I think I ended up seeing about a quarter of game on TV—quite a different experience for a devoted Nebraska fan.

From Laura Janitz
Carrie's Best Friend

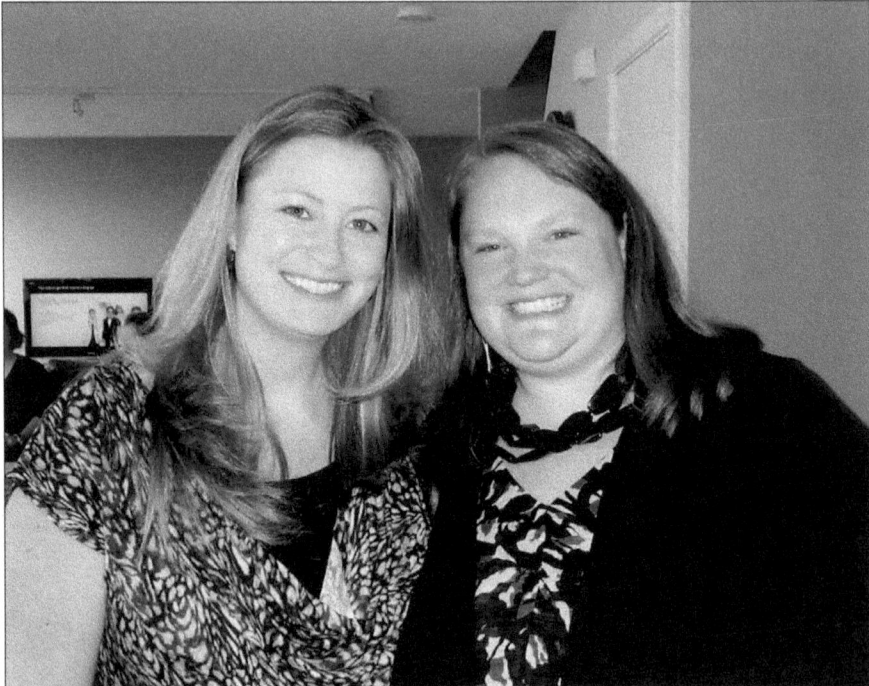

Carrie with her best friend Laura.

I can still remember exactly where I was and what I was doing when I found out Carrie was going into the hospital. I was standing in a Starbucks in downtown Chicago. My husband and then two-year-old daughter were in the car. She had just finished an early morning gymnastics class and we needed coffee to get through the rest of the morning—decaf for me, as I was about four months pregnant with our son.

I was standing in line waiting to order and I got a text from Carrie's husband, Jeff, letting us (our collective group of girlfriends affectionately known as BACH) know that Carrie was still not feeling well and that he was taking her to the hospital. I was confused. She had told us via group text the day before that she thought she had the flu and had gone to the doctor for some meds. I think we all wished her well and a speedy recovery, but no one thought much more of it. Jeff's text caused me to pause.

Later that day, Carrie texted that she still wasn't feeling better, but they'd sent her home from the hospital, thinking she just needed more time to recover. Monday morning we heard from Jeff again. Carrie had woken up unable to move her legs, so he was taking her back to the ER. Jeff was concerned. Jeff is usually the voice of reason in their relationship. If Jeff was concerned, I was concerned. Also, I knew Jeff needed help. Carrie's family lives in Nebraska, and Jeff's family lives in Kansas. They would need someone to watch their three-year-old son, Will, that night.

Jeff kept us posted during the day. He was reading too much Web MD. (What else do you do when you are at the hospital all day?), and sending us all of these crazy ideas of what he thought could be the cause of Carrie's symptoms. Most concerning, though, was that the doctors didn't know what it was either. They were running tests. As the day got later and there were no answers, I told my husband he needed to pick our daughter up from school, and I headed up to Jeff and Carrie's to hang out with Will. I saw Jeff briefly, the worry clear on his face. By this point Carrie's parents were en route from Nebraska. Jeff was planning to stay at the hospital; I was planning to stay with Will until Carrie's parents arrived. Little did I know, this "all hands on deck" approach would shape many of our lives for the next several months

Once Will went to bed, I started Googling Carrie's symptoms and, like Jeff, trying to diagnose her using the internet. When Carrie's dad, Dick Campbell, walked into the house at midnight, before he even said hello, he declared "I think Carrie has Guillain-Barré!" I had come to the same conclusion. We would later find out we were right. But what the hell was Guillain-Barré?

Over the next several days Carrie's condition worsened. By Thursday she was fully paralyzed and eventually needed to be intubated to help her breathe. It was determined that she needed to be taken downtown to Northwestern Memorial's ICU where she would stay through the month.

I remember the first time I saw her in the hospital just a few days later. It was jarring when I walked in to see Carrie laid up in bed covered in wires and tubes, only able to blink. Harder, was not reacting when I saw her. I remember fighting back tears and mentally telling myself to keep it together.

Her parents were there and upbeat (as we were all trying to be for Carrie's sake). They had just mastered a technique to communicate with Carrie. We would hold up a card that had rows of letters. Each row was marked with a number. We would read numbers and when we got to the correct row, she would blink. Then we would name each letter in the row until we got to the correct one and she would blink again. We would repeat this until a word was spelled. Of course as we would get letters, we would try to guess what she was trying to say. So that first day she started to spell out B, and we all guessed bed. "Do you need to bed raised/lowered?"

Shake of the head, then A, then C-K. Back!

"Does your back hurt (she couldn't even feel her back)? Do you need us to back up?"

Then W-A-R-D. Hmmm. Then C-A-R-D. Oh! Backward Card! Yeah, her dad was holding the card with the letters on it backwards. It took a good fifteen minutes to figure that out. We all had a good laugh. Carrie simply rolled her eyes.

After her parents left, she spelled out T-E-L-L M-E S-T-O-R-I-E-S. I thought "there's our girl!" Carrie always loves a good story. The problem was that the only story worth telling at that time was that Carrie was in the hospital with this really weird disease! I tried to do my best.

Not long after her arrival at Northwestern, we decided that due to her not being able to speak, and her friends and family knowing her best, we would have a rotating schedule of people to spend the night with her. Think about it. If you can't talk, and you can't move, how do you alert someone that you need help? She could click her tongue, but a nurse in the hallway couldn't hear that.

The first night I was scheduled to spend the night with her, was a particularly rough day. Jeff had been at the hospital most of the day, along with Carrie's parents and Brooke. Jeff's parents were staying with Will, but Jeff was desperate to get home, sleep in his own bed, and take a shower. He was wiped. When I arrived, it was clear Carrie was not doing well. At this point the disease was continuing to progress and she was uncomfortable.

Her blood pressure was spiking (indicating that she was stressed), so we tried to calm her down by talking about some of her favorite TV shows like *The Bachelor* and *Scandal*. It got to the point where she was going too long in between breaths. The machine in her room was going crazy and we were watching the monitor that showed us when she took a breath. Carrie's mom, Kathy, held Carrie's hand, and very calmly kept saying "Carrie, I need you to take a breath. Great job, now Carrie, I need you to take another breath. Come on Carrie, you need to breathe, breathe Carrie…great job…."

I will never forget that night or that moment, especially as a mother. Here is a woman who is watching her daughter in so much pain and struggling to breathe, and she's not crying, she's just very calmly telling her daughter to *breathe*. I was awestruck. I still am. Ultimately Carrie decided she needed Jeff, so we called him, and he made the hour drive back downtown to be with her.

On my way home, I called our friend Patty who lives in Michigan and wanted regular updates. As I was recounting the night, Patty said, "Is Carrie going to die?!" I honestly couldn't answer. I said no. From what I'd read, people don't die from Guillain-Barré, but at the same time I was thinking about her not being able to breathe. What a night.

Carrie's birthday was December 18th. At this point she'd been in the hospital for at least a week. Carrie loves her birthday, so we did the best we could. We gathered as many people as possible and she had a parade of visitors that day. There were out-of-town visitors, there was cake (that she couldn't eat), there was singing, and then there was a dinner (she obviously didn't attend), where Jeff got himself a much-needed cocktail and we all did a huge toast to Carrie.

At the end of December Carrie was given the good news that she was moving to the Rehabilitation Institute of Chicago (RIC) to continue her recovery. The initial bad news was that she wouldn't be able to have overnight visitors. Carrie was still unable to communicate, and, as the disease was working its way out, her nervous system was all over the place. She would experience hot flashes, cold spells, or need massages, often in the middle of the night. Luckily, with the powers of persuasion we were able to convince the nurses and doctors to let her have one person spend the night. Between Jeff, Brooke, Jen, me, and often a drop-in guest we were able to get all the nights covered.

We got to know the nurses and knew which ones were good, and which weren't, so we'd be on alert at night if we knew we didn't have a good nurse. We watched a lot of *The Bachelor*, and cooking shows, and watched Carrie progress. I remember the first time I walked in and she waved to me. (Yay! She can use her hands!) She had a trach tube and there was a lot of suctioning that needed to occur. I tried unsuccessfully to learn to lip read. Poor Carrie would sometimes just give up if we didn't know what she was trying to say. I think I was mostly able to hear her clicking her tongue to get my attention at night if she needed something. There were a lot of cold wash cloths (she was so hot to the touch, that they wouldn't stay cold very long), and lots of massages as she was experiencing a lot of tingling as feeling was coming back.

During those months that Carrie was in the hospital, lots of people commented to me, and the rest of us, that we were "great friends". Yes, we were, but what I don't think many people understood is that when it comes to being a good friend, Carrie sets the bar. There was never once a feeling of "Ugh, I guess I'll go see Carrie, or I HAVE to go to the RIC tonight." Instead, I was excited to see her, to hear about the progress she was making, and to know that she had the comfort of knowing that someone was there. There was never a question of pitching in to help. It was what Carrie would do.

I've known Carrie for twenty years. We met in college but didn't really become friends until senior year and have stayed friends since. In college I watched as she successfully ran several student organizations while maintaining the grades necessary to graduate with honors, and still found time for frequent social outings. One of my favorite phrases from Carrie was, "Laura, twenty years from now are you going to remember how you did on tomorrow's test or that we went to the Cubs game tonight?" Hard to argue with that point. As I looked at her on graduation day in her gown with her gold honors sash, I was in awe of how she did it all. I am still in awe. Carrie has unsurprisingly become very successful professionally with continued promotions and accolades at work. She is also an amazing mother to (now) two amazing little boys. She finds the time to attend all of her sons' many sporting events, has regular date nights with her husband, (still) attends Cubs games frequently, organizes several vacations a year, has time to share thoughtful comments on every Facebook post of her good friends, and even with all of that, I know that if I needed something, Carrie would be there for me—in a second. That is the true definition of a "good friend", and I am lucky beyond measure to have someone like Carrie in my life.

I hope her story inspires others as it did all of us who were lucky enough to be by her side as she fought her way back to health.

From Jennifer Becker
Carrie's Best Friend

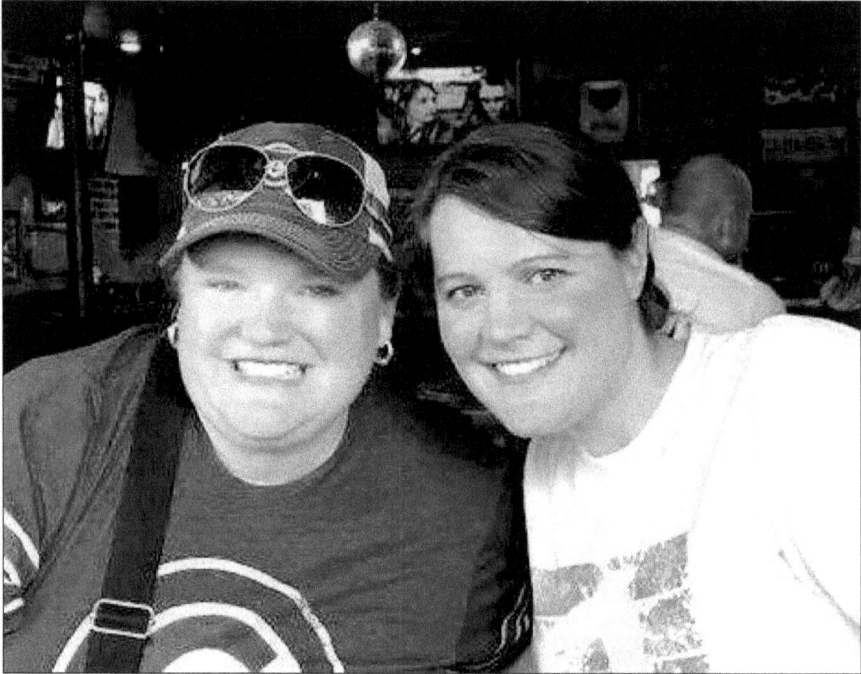

Carrie and her best friend Jennifer.

Memory is a funny thing—what we remember and what we don't. In general, I have a horrible memory. Carrie and I have that in common, though she owns it much better than I do. She might recall a memory that is a shade of an actual event, only to quickly be corrected by one of our friends. Her response is a simple shoulder shrug as if to say, "It is what it is."

I bring up memory and recall because I struggle on the timeline of events during Carrie's journey between December 2013 and September 2014. For lack of a better way to articulate this, my 'memory' falls into two buckets: what I remember and what I don't.

I don't remember the exact moment when I heard Carrie was in trouble. I don't remember who the communication came from. I don't remember if I underplayed the seriousness or was scared to death at the initial description of what was happening.

I do remember going to Northwestern for the first time and being nervous. Nervous driving, nervous parking, and nervous walking in. I think the nervousness was driven by the unknown—would she look better or worse than what I had conjured in my head based on calls and texts from Jeff, Brooke, and Laura Ball who had been there. I'm sure commonalities have emerged as people reflect on the first moment walking into Carrie's hospital room. I assure you that one will be the gut punch of seeing her in the bed with tubes—so many tubes—attached from Carrie to blinking, bleeping machines. This is a memory that will never leave me.

I don't remember who else was in the room when I arrived. I don't remember if they saw the fear that I was experiencing. I doubt they would or should have cared, given their own.

I do remember digging my fingernails into my palm to prevent a complete breakdown when I saw Carrie. Over the course of a couple weeks, so many people entered that room with varying levels of emotion. Every ounce of that emotion was driven by knowing that the person lying in the bed had played a significant role in their life. Carrie had made their lives a little brighter in some way and now they were trying to do the same.

Carrie, you have been one of my best friends for close to eighteen years. You have played numerous roles at differing levels over the years, as happens with friendships. But your ability to provide a sound perspective and a high level of humor has not changed. You can shout out a really insightful comment like, "If you are irreplaceable, you are not promotable." On the flip side, you can make beer come out of my noise by asking "Does beer have bubbles?" or "I don't like bars of soap, they don't get me clean."

I don't remember when the posting and outcry of love and support hit Facebook. I could have looked, but that felt like cheating a little. There was such an immediate response to the updates: offers to help, messages of thoughts and prayers, and, my personal favorite, any mention of a yellow sweat suit.

I do remember hugging Jeff at one point and wanting to hold him a little tighter and a little longer—neither of which would have been comforting enough to release even an ounce of the bundle of confusion, fear, and sadness he was carrying. The load that Jeff carried physically, mentally, and emotionally had to have been back breaking. The resilience Jeff showed over that year was nothing short of amazing. Anyone who was part of this journey was in awe of the husband, son-in-law, and father that he was.

I don't remember when Patty, Laura, Brooke and I first discussed moving back our annual girl's trip, but I do remember the conversation on whether we'd think of it as a cancellation or a postponement, and the emotions during that discussion. (Note: We went on that trip in October 2014 to Saugatuck, Michigan.)

I do remember Carrie blinking through a matrix of letters to spell out entire sentences, and being in such complete confusion at the disconnect between her physical state and her mental state, while having zero concept of her emotional state.

I don't remember the phone call that they had FINALLY hypothesized/figured out her diagnosis.

I do remember Googling Guillain-Barré syndrome (of course, I spelled it wrong the first time) for hours, going down the rabbit hole of medical opinions, treatments, and patient stories. Feeling a sense of relief that FINALLY there was something tangible to be done and while the road ahead was very long, Carrie and Jeff could actually envision that there was a road. I also remember being so impressed with Brooke's level of knowledge compared to mine... even with all my Googling.

I don't remember when Carrie was transferred from the ICU to the rehab center.

I do remember being sound asleep in what can only be described as a freezer disguised as a hospital room, when I was abruptly awakened by a flurry of activity. That was the night I thought things had taken a turn... for the worse.

I don't remember exactly what had happened, but I remember being scared for Carrie as I left that next morning, even though she was good when I left.

I do remember feeling insecure about my inability to keep up a good, long conversation with myself (because Carrie could not verbally respond) as well as Laura Ball and Bridget. I tried really hard to add additional details to stories in an effort to "compete." I kept thinking, "Would Carrie rather have someone longer winded than me here?"

I don't remember if it was allowed or illegal, but we ate Chinese food in the rehab center, then laughed about how we were eating Chinese food in the rehab center.

I don't remember Carrie's official release date.

I do remember an image of Carrie outside with a walker in a tee-shirt and shorts before leaving to go home. Maybe another Facebook memory?

I don't remember the timing lag from when Carrie was released to when she had to go back to get her throat tube (100 percent positive that is not the name) out.

I do remember that Carrie's release was just a chapter but not the end of her journey.

I am reminded often of the impact of this chapter on Carrie's journey. Reminded by the perspective she now has on life and balance. Reminded when I see pictures of the Grimes or Campbell families. Reminded when Carrie calls for a rest break when hiking because she knows her physical limits. Reminded when I see an invite pop up from Carrie for a Barn Dance or a half-birthday celebration. Reminded when I see the way Carrie looks at Jeff or Will or Zach.

We are lucky to be a part of your journey Carrie, and lucky that you are a part of ours.

From Kathy Campbell
Carrie's Mom

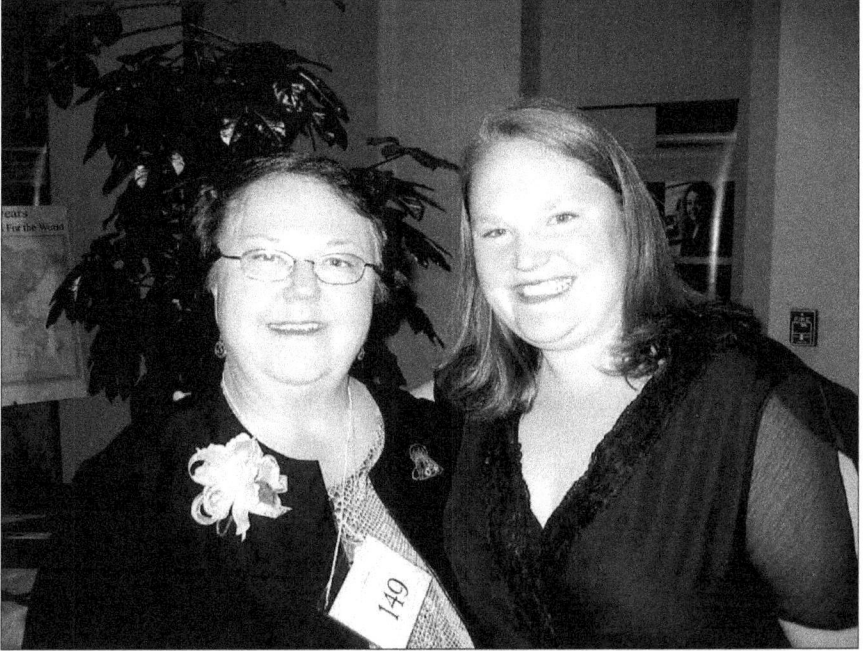

Carrie and her Mother, Kathy.

People continue to ask about Carrie. How is she doing, did she fully recover? My response: Every morning I wake up I know I am blessed! In our lives, we experience many blessings, but none so profoundly impactful as Carrie's journey to full recovery from GBS.

I often quipped that I was going to title my section "80 on 80"—frantically driving the I-80 roadway to Chicago that December night. It was just surreal! Listening to Christmas carols, watching the sparkling lights on the Christmas trees of farmsteads, mentally making a list of presents for Will. Periodic calls during the trip from Jeff and Carrie: No answers yet, the paralysis continues creeping upward. And in Carrie's voice, hearing how scary this truly was as she asked for prayers.

Through the next year, faith and prayers from so many people were powerful, encouraging, and a sustaining support. But Carrie's faith, tenacity, work ethic and determined spirit as well as Jeff's unfailing love were the encouragements I held in my heart. Protecting your children and doing what it takes to make it all better, is at the core of parenthood. In the first weeks, I felt helpless and fearful of losing her or what life-altering physical challenges were ahead. I just wanted to take her in my arms. How could this be happening? But as the parent, you smile, reassure, and believe God is with her. And you find hope in every sign of recovery.

And in this time, we gathered wonderful memories …watching Will in his excitement on Christmas morning, playing games with him each time we drove to the hospital, and watching his love for Mom as he lie beside her. And for that year, we also found the joy in simple moments: Dick and I enjoying a very romantic New Year's Eve dinner in the parking lot of the downtown Chicago McDonald's in the midst of a snowstorm. Hearing Carrie's voice in her first phone call to me. Will surprising his mom as Spider-Man. And the joy of seeing this highly competitive young woman exceed the weekly goals.

The most difficult periods of 2014 for me were leaving Carrie. After spending most of December in Libertyville/Chicago, Dick, Andy and I were to return to Lincoln in early January. Carrie had transitioned to RIC and there were signs of improvement. The Nebraska Legislature was about to convene. As a State Senator I had major legislation to introduce, most notably, a bill to expand Medicaid for low income Nebraskans. But saying goodbye to Carrie was heartbreaking. There were so many days, sitting in the legislative chamber, that I almost left for Chicago. But my staff, fellow Senators, and people throughout the Capitol were a constant support. And, almost every day, we'd hear of prayer chains springing up across the country in every religion for Carrie, enveloping her and all of us.

Each month either Dick, Andy, or I visited, and each time, progress was very evident. From pushing small sponges from one hand to the other, "driving" her wheelchair, standing, and eventually walking out of RIC to go home, each milestone represented hours of painstaking effort. We'd try to be helpful during our visits. Andy walked to McDonalds to get his sister fries and a fountain Coke during the worst cold spell in Chicago history. I, however, failed in the role of hairdresser. Carrie's PT therapist walked in the day room, "Who did your hair? It's horrible!" Not only was the physical progress encouraging, but just being together, playing games, and meeting her therapists and care givers helped us see the Carrie we loved returning. It was the sure sign of hope.

At the end of the legislative session, I spent two and half months with Carrie, Jeff, and Will during her out-patient recovery. I am sure I benefited from this experience far more than my help benefited them. To spend an extended time with my daughter was a gift—laughing, sharing memories and being a part of their daily lives. And I shall always remember and cherish spending time with Will. Every night we'd go to my room and read a book or two and talk. But on a special evening, he went to his first Cubs baseball game with his parents for his birthday present. I heard them arrive home, the back door thrown open, and his voice, "Mimi, Mimi, Mimi—where are you?" He came running up the stairs and into my room. "I had the best time! I'm going to go every single day!" A moment of sheer joy!

In 2014, there were not many moments of sheer joy—for Carrie, perhaps more moments of pain, suffering, and setbacks. But her story is not to be remembered for the many struggles, but for her indominable spirit and faith to believe she would recover, and for the courage to persevere.

"There is in every true woman's heart, a spark of heavenly fire, which lies dormant in the broad daylight of prosperity, but which kindles up and beams and blazes in the dark hour of adversity."

-Washington Irving

The following article about Kathy's journey with Carrie appeared in the *Lincoln Journal* on April 20, 2014.

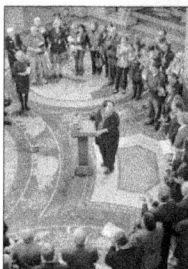

Senator got front-row view of health issues

By JoANNE YOUNG
Lincoln Journal Star

The call came on Dec. 9, halting Lincoln Sen. Kathy Campbell's jam-packed day.

A month before the legislative session, she was knee-deep in talks with staff and senators about a controversial bill she would introduce to expand Medicaid to about 60,000 Nebraska adults as allowed by the Affordable Care Act.

The bill had resistance, not only from Gov. Dave Heineman but a faction of senators who had filibustered it in 2013.

The call from her son-in-law would give her a personal context for her work, sending her on a health-care journey with her daughter, Carrie Grimes, who lives eight hours away in Chicago. She would see close up how quickly the need for good medical insurance can descend on a family.

Campbell's daughter had been admitted to the intensive care unit at a Chicago hospital that day with symptoms of tingling in her fingers and feet, and numbness in her lower legs.

"I said, 'Jeff do you want us to come?' and he said 'Yes ... we just don't know what this is. We're very scared about what's happening here,'" Campbell recounted.

Campbell wrapped up what she could on short notice. She and her husband, Dick, jumped in the car that afternoon. As they made their way to their daughter, the numbness crept toward Carrie's knees. By the next morning, it had reached her upper legs.

Doctors confirmed that next day that Carrie had contracted Guillain-Barre syndrome, a fairly rare disorder in which the body's immune system attacks part of the peripheral nervous system and can lead to paralysis.

In Carrie's case, the numbness would progress to her upper body and would affect her ability to breathe, swallow and talk.

See SENATOR, Page A2

Sen. Kathy Campbell turns to acknowledge applause from supporters as she joined other state senators and health care advocates during a March rally to push for Medicaid expansion in Nebraska.

Session gave perspective to returning senators

The legislative landscape will change significantly next year. But after fall elections, as many as 32 senators, each with a different perspective and experience, will return for the 104th Legislature that begins in January. Three of them — Lincoln Sen. Kathy Campbell and Omaha Sens. Tanya Cook and Heath Mello — will be among a dozen with six years of experience and seniority. This is what they've learned about leading the state forward.
Monday: Omaha Sen. Tanya Cook is a unique role model for the Legislature.
Tuesday: Appropriations Chairman Heath Mello led senators through a thorny state budget.

Senator got front-row view of health issues
By JoAnne Young

The call came on Dec. 9, halting Lincoln Sen. Kathy Campbell's jam-packed day.

A month before the legislative session, she was knee-deep in talk with staff and senators about a controversial bill she would introduce to expand Medicaid to about 60,000 Nebraska adults as allowed by the Affordable Care Act.

The bill has resistance, not only from Gov. Dave Heineman but a faction of senators who had filibustered it in 2013.

317

The call from her son-in-law would give her a personal context for her work, sending her on a health-care journey with her daughter Carrie Grimes, who lives eight hours away in Chicago. She would see close up how quickly the need for good medical insurance can descend on a family.

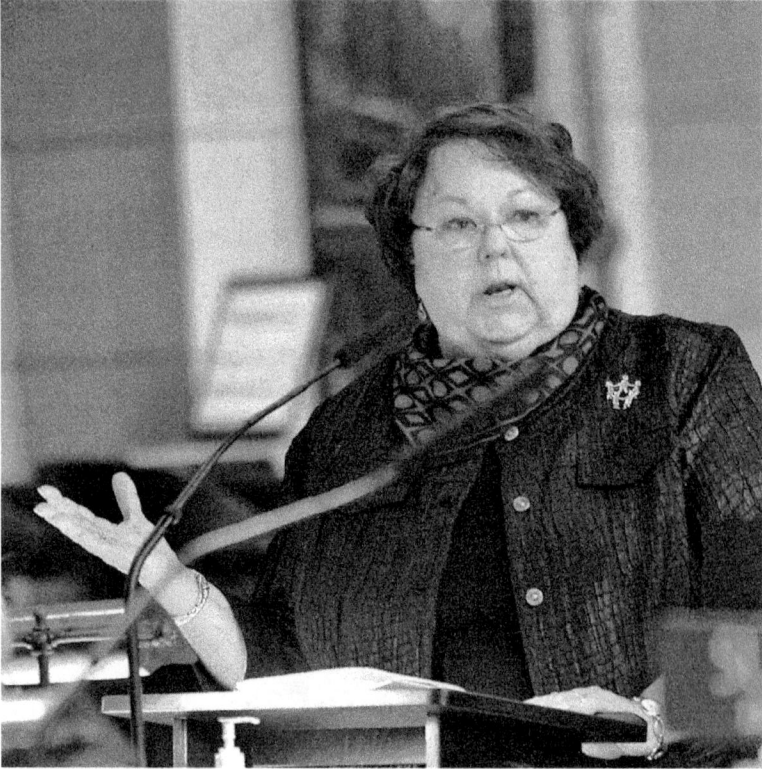

Kathy, Carrie's mom, introducing Children's Health and Welfare bills as Chair of the Health and Human Services Committee.

Campbell's daughter had been admitted to the intensive care unit at a Chicago hospital that day with symptoms of tingling in her fingers and feet, and numbness in her lower legs.

"I said, 'Jeff do you want us to come?' and he said, 'Yes ... we just don't know what this is. We're very scared about what's happening here,'" Campbell recounted.

Campbell wrapped up what she could on short notice. She and her husband, Dick, jumped in the car that afternoon. As they made their way to their daughter, the numbness crept toward Carrie's knees. By the next morning, it had reached her upper legs.

Doctors confirmed that next day that Carrie had contracted Guillain-Barre syndrome, a fairly rare disorder in which the body's immune system attacks part of the peripheral nervous system and can lead to paralysis.

In Carrie's case, the numbness would progress to her upper body and would affect her ability to breathe, swallow and talk.

People with Guillain-Barre usually recover fully, but there was at least one night in the first week when Carrie's breaths were getting shorter, and shallower, that Campbell wasn't sure what the outcome would be.

"That was kind of a long night because it just seemed like every monitor was going off," she said.

A couple of days later, Campbell had to return to Lincoln to attend a hearing on Medicaid expansion at the Capitol. Then two days later, they packed up and returned to Chicago to look after their 3-year-old grandson and help with Christmas.

Throughout December, Campbell had relied on her staff, especially committee attorney Michelle Chaffee, to refine the bill Campbell would introduce in the early days of the year's session: the Wellness in Nebraska Act (LB887) that would expand Medicaid to tens of thousands of state residents.

"I really think that Carrie's experience underscored for me the need for WIN because I kept thinking, 'What if Carrie and Jeff had no insurance?'" Campbell said.

They both had good jobs. But Campbell questions how differently things would have gone without insurance, how much recovery help Carrie would have received and how much they would have had to spend of their own resources.

The first three days in ICU was $155,000, she said. What would four months of hospital charges and rehabilitation cost?

On Dec. 27, after 18 days in the intensive care unit, Carrie was released to a rehabilitation hospital to start her recovery. The progression of the syndrome and paralysis had stabilized, stopping at her neck.

On Jan. 4, Campbell drove back to Lincoln for the start of the session.

"That was a really long ride for me because I just kept thinking, 'Should I say in Chicago?'" She said.

A lot of things fell into place, Campbell said, that made it OK for her to be in Lincoln. But she was distracted at times and felt more distant from the lawmaking process. She introduced only a few bills and attended very few events.

She traveled back to Chicago during two four-day recesses of the Legislature in February and March. And she tried to email Carrie daily.

By Feb. 13, Carrie was off a ventilator. By the March recess, she was relearning to walk. On April 2, she was able to go home, to walk with the help of a walker and attend daylong outpatient therapies.

It put things into perspective for Campbell, especially when senators spent hours at the Capitol debating bills with narrow impact.

"I have to say, and I know it was very important to some people, that the days we spent on the flashing yellow lights (LB399) is when I (said to myself), 'You know, maybe I shouldn't be here. Maybe I should go back to Chicago,'" she said.

As Campbell worked on Medicaid, she pondered every email she got from uninsured people who talked about serious health problems, who had gone without proper diagnosis and adequate medication.

"It made it a whole lot more personal, that's probably No. 1," she said. "I think I was certainly far more empathetic to all the people who wrote me. ... I could have spent my whole time on the floor just reading emails from people."

Campbell was disappointed when a filibuster stopped the bill from getting an up-or-down vote.

But her front-row seat on the issue made her more determined to continue to work for those Nebraskans without insurance.

She headed back to Chicago after the session ended last week and will focus her time for a while on helping her daughter in the weeks ahead.

And she'll mull over her plans for next year's session. A lot of health and child welfare issues still need close attention.

The Wellness in Nebraska Act "is great health policy," she said. "We have to do a better job of saying to our neighbors, 'you know this is important. ... We spend a lot of time trying to talk to senators, but to some extent, I think we've got to talk to Nebraskans."

From Jeff Grimes
Carrie's Husband

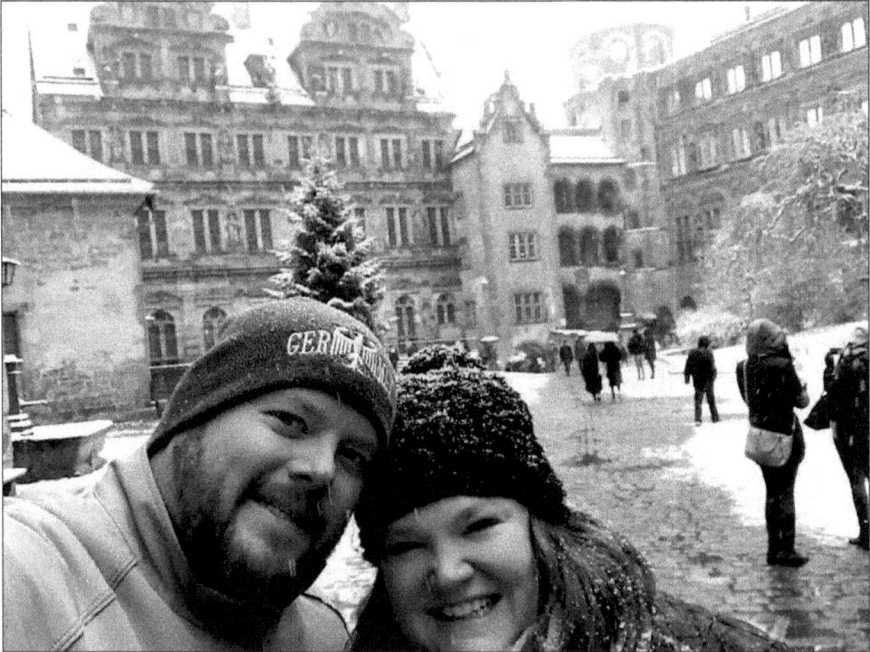

Jeff and Carrie traveling in Germany together – enjoying life post GBS.

Carrie has asked me over and over to write something down about my experiences while we went through the single most stressful, frustrating, and terrifying situation we've ever dealt with. You've read my emails in this book and Carrie has provided a lot of the additional details of her journey with GBS. What I never really talked about were my personal feelings and struggle with all of it. I have sat down countless times to write this over the last several years, and every time I'd start to recall I got so emotional it halted my ability to write.

The first thing I remember every time is fear. Fear that we didn't know what was going on for days. Fear that Carrie was going to die, and I would be left with a little boy, a house we'd just bought in a place where we have very little family support. Fear that she would never come off the ventilator. Fear that she would never walk again. Fear that her trachea was permanently damaged and she would be on a breathing apparatus for the rest of her life. Fear that Will was going to grow up without a mom, or with a mom with very limited physical capability.

One problem I recognized very early in the process is something I'd known at a low level for a long time. Carrie is an absolute extrovert—she feeds off of the energy she's given. If she is given bad news, poor feedback, or even has an unexpected argument, Carrie will immediately begin to doubt, question, and internalize. If someone is upbeat, positive or has a good report, Carrie is energized and positive. This has held true her entire life and was never more evident than during her ordeal with GBS.

Very early in this nightmare year, I was having a discussion with one of the doctors at Lake Forest who, every single time we spoke with him, gave us the worst possible prognosis for

Carrie's case. The second day I followed him out of the room and asked what I would eventually ask every health care professional, friend, and visitor who interacted with Carrie: "Please try to be as positive and encouraging as possible around her. If you have truly bad news, please consider the impact or let me tell her so I can make it less stressful for her."

While we were in Lake Forest, I could see all of the bad news hitting Carrie like punches to the gut. She was already physically beaten up and every bad reports came like a mental blow, multiple times a day. The day we moved from Lake Forest to Chicago was one of the roughest—the ambulance problems, the breathing issues, and her mental state all deteriorating rapidly. I honestly think the reason she was put on such a high dose of Propofol wasn't because of the GBS, it was because she was so scared and worried about the entire prognosis from the doctors and nurses. We saw a change at RIC, with all of her physical and occupational therapists. By nature, most of them were absolutely, relentlessly positive and I never had to do anything but encourage her while she was in PT or OT. The first few weeks, when even moving a single muscle was a good sign, all of the therapists were her cheering section, and it absolutely motivated her to keep working and get better, even though every day she had massive nerve pain, cold and hot spells, and complete physical exhaustion as her body recovered from its trauma.

The second thing I remember is my own exhaustion. The first week I tried to go home three times to get a shower and sleep. Each time, Carrie was upset or in distress and I went right back. Sleeping in a chair in an ICU room is not fun for one day, much less weeks at a time. I would be with Carrie all day, going to appointments, going to therapies, talking to doctors, talking to friends and visitors, and then at night try to catch up with parents, Will, email, and some work. Once we were able to establish a routine at RIC, her girlfriends would help me by giving a couple overnights a week to go home, shower, get clean clothes and see Will. I remember multiple times hearing, "Daddy, wake up!" from Will after I fell asleep playing LEGO, or reading books on these short breaks. Once Carrie progressed further in recovery and started getting off the ventilator, RIC moved her into a double room, where I could no longer spend the night with her. I would then go to Brooke and Jeff's house and pass out in their guest bedroom. I tried once or twice to make conversation or watch a bit of TV, but generally it would be shower, sleep and back to RIC the next morning. I will never be able to thank Brooke and Jeff enough for their kindness and generosity in letting me camp in their spare room for literally months while Carrie was at RIC, along with Brooke's weekly and often twice weekly visits and overnights with Carrie.

The third thing I remember is being so thankful for both sets of parents and what seemed to be the endless legion of people who loved and cared about Carrie so much they would do whatever they could to help. Both Carrie's and my parents spent weeks, if not months, during one of the coldest winters in recent history taking care of the house, keeping Will on his regular schedule of daycare, gymnastics and swimming, and visiting her as often as possible. I could not have spent all of the time that I did with Carrie if they had not dropped everything to help us. I could also not have survived without Carrie's best girlfriends setting up a rotation of staying overnight with her when I was worn down. Brooke, Laura, and Jen were absolute angels, and Patty and Stephanie always buoyed Carrie when they could come. The other people who helped by visiting, sending flowers, emails, phone calls were helpful beyond measure because they again reinforced the positive mindset that was absolutely the primary factor in Carrie's recovery. I'm pretty sure I also owe friends several apologies because the once or twice I was able to join them for birthday celebrations or similar events, I was either maudlin, very quickly inebriated, or both.

Once the madness of December and January subsided, the thing I will always remember most is my worry for Will. At three, I was never really sure how much he understood about what was going on. The first few times he visited Carrie in the hospital she had tubes and monitors and he was just overwhelmed. He buried his head in my shoulder and was scared to even touch Mommy. I finally got him to give her a kiss and that lit her eyes up for the first time in days. When Mimi and Papa or Grammy and Grandad would bring him down to visit, he was always so excited to see Mommy, play with doctor gloves, and talk to Mommy about school. When I would come home, he would be so excited to see me and so upset when I would leave to go back to Carrie. There were a lot of LEGO and donut bribes that winter, but even then, he really struggled with gymnastics and swimming without Carrie and me there. Thankfully, he doesn't seem to remember much of it, other than Carrie was in the hospital and he got lots of blue gloves.

The last major memories I have are conflicting. I was so relieved that Carrie was finally on the road to recovery. In February alone she started to come off the ventilator, stood up without a harness, started gaining strength in hands and feet, and many more amazing milestones. All of that was tempered by the fact that on a daily basis we were surrounded by people who were likely at the furthest point of their recovery and would be in wheelchairs or using assisting devices for the rest of their lives. It was a daily struggle for Carrie to remain positive when surrounded by a lot of folks dealing with injuries or illnesses that would permanently change their quality of life. More than once I heard from other people that they were so glad Carrie was on their floor because she was so positive about her situation and her therapy, but it was also hard for them and their families because their own rehab was not progressing like hers.

The most lasting lesson I have from Carrie's GBS journey was something I had heard before but never expected to experience until much later in life. The biggest struggle for me outside of all the mental and emotional struggles was the medical experience itself. The doctors, nurses, assistants, therapists, and insurance people all have their own opinions, but it is absolutely critical that you and your family do the best you possibly can to advocate for your own health. Multiple times we had issues with doctors waffling on decisions, nurses not following procedures, therapists giving conflicting advice, and the largest issue—the post-ventilator tracheal drama. I had so many conversations with the ENT's PA I'm pretty sure she started call screening me and dumping me to voicemail after a while. I also had argument after argument with the RIC patient advocate, her health insurance adjusters and doctors, and her job HR and benefits teams. I am not and have never been an aggressive person (as Carrie can confirm), but for her sake I had to make sure she was getting the best possible care and benefits she could during this journey.

While I'd like to hope no one would ever have to go through the ordeal that Carrie did, I know it happens every day to someone. The best advice I can give is to always try to stay positive for yourself and others, take care of yourself as a caregiver too, be thankful for friends and family and be the biggest and best advocate for medical care as you possibly can.

I love you Caroline.

www.ingramcontent.com/pod-product-compliance
Lightning Source LLC
Chambersburg PA
CBHW072049020426
42334CB00017B/1448